Intermittent Fasting for Women over 50 Mastery

A Proven Method for Weight Loss after Menopause, Anti-aging and Longevity

Paul Griggs

Your FREE Book Bonus!

Thank you so much for your purchase! Here is a free gift to help implement the recommendations in this book. Inside, you will find delicious healthy recipes for appetizers, lunch and dinner, with foods for your hormones to complement your fasting lifestyle.

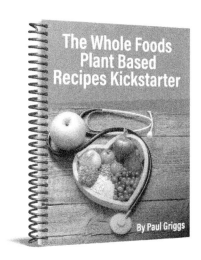

Get your free book bonus here:

paulgriggs.aweb.page/kickstarterIF

Contents

Introduction

Fasting is completely different from diets that tell you what to do. Many diets focus on what to eat, but intermittent fasting is all about when you eat. It doesn't tell you what to do, it tells you what not to do. And unlike many other interventions, it's free.

- *Jason Fung, MD, nephrologist, bestselling author of The Obesity Code*

As women navigate through the transformative years following menopause, they experience significant changes like weight gain, hormonal imbalance, reduced mental performance, and overall health. This book is for you: women over 50. The purpose of this book is to empower and inspire postmenopausal women to embrace intermittent fasting for improved weight, self-image, health, and longevity.

If you answer yes to any of these questions, this book is for you:

1. Are you a woman over 50 who wants lasting abdominal fat loss? Without changing diet or exercise?
2. Would you like to lose weight in a way that is shown to prevent and improve diseases like diabetes, high blood pressure, high cholesterol, and metabolic syndrome?
3. Do you want to lose weight while lowering your risk for cancer?
4. Do you want to boost your energy and balance your hormones for peak performance?

5. Do you want to improve your mood, anxiety, mental clarity, and memory? Using the same method shown to reduce your risk of Alzheimer's / dementia?
6. Do you want a customizable plan to help you change when you eat to suit your goals and lifestyle? A plan based on real results achieved by women just like you?

Leading scientific research shows lasting weight loss is one of many benefits of fasting. Intermittent fasting is simply structured eating; not eating for a specified period of time each day. In this book you will learn the science of intermittent fasting, all the reasons to do it, and how to do it. You will discover how to do this using clinically proven methods for postmenopausal women leveraging the miracle that is human physiology, refined over eons of evolution.

The most important thing when learning is credibility. Before you can teach, you must know. Please note the wisdom that follows is not coming from me. It is found in decades of scientific literature and comes from three world-renowned fasting authorities: Dr. Fung, Dr. Longo, and Dr. Mattson. Dr. Jason Fung is a lecturer to physicians on fasting, weight loss and reversing diabetes, bestselling author of *The Obesity Code*, and founder of The Fasting Method clinic. He may be the highest clinical authority on fasting and weight loss. You will be hearing from Dr. Fung throughout this book. You will also hear from Dr. Longo, Director of the Longevity Institute, a leader in age-related disease and creator of the fasting-mimicking diet. He has researched fasting, anti-aging, and longevity for over 30 years. You will also hear from Dr. Mattson, a fasting researcher for over 20 years and colleague of Dr. Longo.

How will intermittent fasting help me?

In 2019 the prestigious *New England Journal of Medicine* reviewed the health benefits of intermittent fasting beyond abdominal fat loss: decreasing inflammation, blood sugar, blood pressure, and lower risk of diabetes and cancer.[1] In this research review, Dr. Mattson said it best:

> Intermittent fasting elicits evolutionarily conserved, adaptive cellular responses in a manner that improves glucose regulation, increases stress resistance, and suppresses inflammation. During fasting, cells activate pathways that enhance intrinsic defenses against oxidative stress... During the feeding period, cells engage in tissue-specific processes of growth and [healing]. However, most people consume three meals a day plus snacks, so intermittent fasting does not occur.[2]

Dr. Mattson is saying fasting activates natural healing mechanisms that repair damage and promote growth. The problem is that people eat too many hours a day to enjoy these benefits. Intermittent fasting decreases the number of eating hours per day.

There are virtually countless benefits of intermittent fasting. It has been shown to lose weight long term, enhance mental performance, balance hormones, lower cancer risk, improve cardiovascular health, slow aging, and increase lifespan. By harnessing these benefits, women over 50 can embrace intermittent fasting as a powerful tool to not only transform

[1] De Cabo R, Mattson MP. Effects of intermittent fasting on health, aging, and disease. *The New England Journal of Medicine*. 2019;381(26):2541-2551. doi:10.1056/nejmra1905136
[2] Ibid.

their physical appearance but improve their quality of life and lifespan.

Intermittent fasting myths

Before moving on to Chapter 1, let's address some of the common objections and myths about intermittent fasting. One big reason there are thousands of success stories with fasting is that it does not require time or money.

Myth 1: Fasting won't work for weight loss.

If you don't eat, do you really think you will not lose weight? You will. The truth is in the coming chapters.

Myth 2: Fasting is too expensive.

Actually, fasting does not cost you more. It doesn't cost more because it doesn't require you to change what you eat. If you don't eat meat, you can fast. If you don't eat wheat, you can fast. If you have a nut allergy, you can fast. If you cook or don't cook, you can fast. Fasting is free and compatible with every diet.

Myth 3: I don't have time to fast.

Fasting saves time. If you don't eat, there's no going out to get food, no grocery shopping, no cooking, and no clean up. Since the eating does not occur it does not take any time. If you travel all the time, you can fast. Everyone has time for fasting because it costs no time.

Myth 4: Fasting will put you into starvation mode and make you gain weight.

In a study of four straight days of fasting, the metabolic rate increased by over 10%.[3] This is the opposite of weight gain. The study showed metabolic rate increased over one to four days of fasting. It follows from human evolution that you burn more calories of fat when fasting as this is how we had the energy to hunt and gather food when food was scarce. Cavemen did not have abundant access to food.

With calorie counting every day your metabolism goes down because you're decreasing calories without changing insulin. Insulin levels go up when you eat, signaling the body to store energy as fat (see Chapter 1). Insulin stays high when you eat every four hours or less, e.g. breakfast, lunch, dinner, snack after dinner. Insulin levels drop when you fast. So what promotes weight gain from starvation mode is calorie counting, not fasting.

To gain weight fasting, with the resulting increased metabolism, you would have to eat **way more** calories than normal when refeeding. Is that what happens? No. A 2002 study showed fasting as long as 36 hours "did not yield a powerful stimulus to compensate the next day."[4] This means fasting does not cause overeating when you resume eating. So it's physiologically impossible to gain weight fasting. Fasting is the way your body burns fat based on eons of evolution.

Myth 5: Fasting causes raging hunger.

---

[3] Zaunder C, et al. Resting energy expenditure in short-term starvation is increased as a result of an increase in serum norepinephrine. *The American Journal of Clinical Nutrition*. 2000;71(6):1511-1515. doi:10.1093/ajcn/71.6.1511

[4] Johnstone AM, et al. Effect of an acute fast on energy compensation and feeding behaviour in lean men and women. *International Journal of Obesity*. 2002;26(12):1623-1628. doi:10.1038/sj.ijo.0802151

Many people believe they'll be too hungry if they don't eat. Research on the human hunger hormone (ghrelin) shows that if you fast by skipping lunch, the hunger hormone drops to zero by 4pm as if you ate lunch.[5] Let me repeat that for emphasis: **whether you eat lunch or not the hunger hormone levels are near zero by 4pm.** The same study shows if you skip dinner, hunger goes up initially but it's back down to zero before midnight whether you ate dinner or not. How is that? The body simply burns stored energy so the hunger disappears.

You can think of your body like a hybrid car. The car can run using electricity or gas. Your body can run on stored sugar or fat.

If fasting causes raging hunger, how come you don't wake up ravenous every day? The same study showed ghrelin levels are near zero from 12am to 7am. That's because you are burning stored energy while you sleep for body heat, circulation, breathing, etc. Since hunger hormone levels are near zero while you sleep you do not wake up hungry after seven hours of not eating.

Moreover, a 2023 review of 23 studies showed intermittent fasting does not increase hunger more than calorie counting.[6] All studies found intermittent fasting is safe and is not associated with feeling hungry to the point participants

---

[5] See Figure 2 in Natalucci G, et al. Spontaneous 24-h ghrelin secretion pattern in fasting subjects: maintenance of a meal-related pattern. *European Journal of Endocrinology.* 2005;152(6):845-850. doi:10.1530/eje.1.01919

[6] Elsworth RL, et al. The Effect of Intermittent Fasting on Appetite: A Systematic Review and Meta-Analysis. Nutrients. 2023 Jun 1;15(11):2604. doi: 10.3390/nu15112604.

stop fasting.[7] This means fasting is sustainable because it is NOT associated with hunger, unlike calorie counting.

Myth 6: Fasting burns muscle.

Jason Fung, MD, is a renowned expert and bestselling author on fasting. Here is Dr. Fung's response to this myth from a 2016 lecture on weight loss:

> Protein is not a storage form of energy. Why would your body burn it for energy? [This argument you're going to burn muscle] is ridiculous... because you're telling me that the way we're designed is to store energy as fat, but when the chips are down we'll burn muscle?[8] It's sort of like storing firewood and instead of burning firewood for heat you throw the sofa in the fire... It makes no sense from a physiologic standpoint and we know from our studies of physiology there's a very, very short period of protein burning, not muscle... As your body doesn't eat it's going to look for a source of calories and take it from the body fat [your abundant stored calories].[9]

A 1983 study showed fasting does not increase protein digestion; the nitrogen waste from protein excreted as urine is lower when fasting.[10] This means when fasting you conserve protein. We do not burn muscle (protein) as fuel.

[7] Ibid

[8] Jason Fung. Fasting and Weight Loss - Solving the Two-Compartment problem. *YouTube*. Published online March 15, 2016. https://www.youtube.com/watch?v=ETkwZIi3R7w at 18:00

[9] Jason Fung. Intermittent Fasting Myths - Top 5 | Intermittent Fasting | Jason Fung. *YouTube*. Published online January 24, 2023. https://www.youtube.com/watch?v=MLxwtwYPkHU at 4:55 − 5:57

[10] Cahill GF Jr. President's address. Starvation. Trans Am Clin Climatol Assoc. 1983;94:1-21. PMID: 6764569

How could we have survived as a species if we burned away our muscle (protein) when we needed to hunt and gather food during famines?

A 2010 study of 70 days of alternate-day fasting showed zero lean muscle loss. [11] It actually showed a slight increase in lean muscle. In 2023 **a review of 48 studies on muscle mass in people over 55 showed fasting two days a week preserved lean muscle** (5:2).[12] It found "the most effective strategy for loss of fat while maintaining or increasing muscle mass was the combination of energy restriction [fasting] and exercise." While the authors use the term "energy restriction" (eating less) in this statement, with 5:2 fasting you have energy restriction two days a week. Since intermittent fasting restricts the window of time to eat it can result in eating less and preserving muscle.

A 2020 review of eight studies found intermittent fasting paired with exercise maintains lean muscle.[13] This review included studies of time-restricted feeding and alternate-day feeding. Moreover, one 2016 study of **16:8 fasting showed an increase in lean muscle**.[14] Research shows

---

[11] See Table 2 in Bhutani S, et al. Improvements in coronary heart disease risk indicators by Alternate-Day Fasting involve adipose tissue modulations. *Obesity*. 2010;18(11):2152-2159. doi:10.1038/oby.2010.54

[12] See Figure 3B Muscle Mass results in Eglseer D, et al. Nutrition and Exercise Interventions to Improve Body Composition for Persons with Overweight or Obesity Near Retirement Age: A Systematic Review and Network Meta-Analysis of Randomized Controlled Trials. *Advances in Nutrition*. 2023;14(3):516-538. doi:10.1016/j.advnut.2023.04.001

[13] Keenan S, Cooke MB, Belski R. The Effects of Intermittent Fasting Combined with Resistance Training on Lean Body Mass: A Systematic Review of Human Studies. Nutrients. 2020 Aug 6;12(8):2349. doi: 10.3390/nu12082349.

[14] Moro T., et al. Effects of eight weeks of time-restricted feeding (16/8) on basal metabolism, maximal strength, body composition,

intermittent fasting does *not* burn muscle, as Dr. Fung tells us.

These are the most common myths and objections about fasting. You can see they have no legs to stand on. I'm not here to tell you fasting is easy. How easy it will be will vary for each person, and it is more complicated for women. However, there are countless fasting methods that can help anyone.

Throughout the pages of this book, we will take a deep dive into intermittent fasting for women over 50, exploring proven strategies, practical tips, and leading scientific research. Whether you are new to intermittent fasting or have prior experience, this book will serve as a comprehensive resource to guide you on your journey towards optimal weight and countless other benefits.

Part I of this book will explain the science of intermittent fasting, and the secret of why it works for losing fat and keeping the weight off. You will also discover countless reasons to fast after menopause, including hormone balancing, mental health, physical health, and anti-aging benefits. Knowing compelling reasons why to fast is key to success.

Part II will show you real women getting real results with weight loss using intermittent fasting and define the proven fasting methods. It will also simplify nutrition for hormone balancing and weight loss. Part III will give you proven,

inflammation, and cardiovascular risk factors in resistance-trained males. J. Transl. Med. 2016;14:290. doi: 10.1186/s12967-016-1044-0.

customizable, weekly fasting plans for weight loss, tips to succeed, and other insights to speed up your results.

Part 1: The Science of Intermittent Fasting for Women

Chapter 1

It's Not Your Fault Trendy Diets Failed

If you say eat 500 calories less a day and you'll lose 1 lb a week, does that mean if you're 200 lbs after 200 weeks you'll weigh zero? Obviously not. You're not going to lose weight until you die. The body has to adapt. This is basic homeostasis. [15]

- *Jason Fung, MD in lecture to other physicians on fasting and weight loss, bestselling author of The Obesity Code*

Before diving into fat burning science, let me ask a few questions to see if they resonate with you. Are you frustrated with yo-yo dieting? Have you tried to mimic another woman's weight loss strategy only to come up short? Are you tired of counting calories, leaving you feeling cold, tired, and hungry? Have you had a doctor say you must lower your BMI for your health without telling you exactly how?

Many women get frustrated and disappointed with trendy diets that promise quick and dramatic weight loss. While these diets may lead to initial weight loss, they ultimately lead to gaining the weight back. Here are some reasons why.

One reason is the emphasis on short term results rather than long term lifestyle changes. Many trending diets adopt an

---

[15] Jason Fung. Science of Intermittent Fasting | Intermittent Fasting | Jason Fung. *YouTube*. Published online July 17, 2022. https://www.youtube.com/watch?v=6aiR1mFD7Gw at 7:27

overly restrictive approach that may lead to rapid weight loss initially. These diets often involve severe calorie counting, restricting entire food groups like carb counting, or reliance on overly processed "diet" products. Such restrictive approaches are difficult to maintain, leading to feelings of deprivation, decreased adherence, and rebound weight gain.

Do you know any women struggling with yo-yo dieting? **Research shows multiple cycles of weight loss (from 7% - 10%) and weight regain are associated with increased mortality.**[16] This means you should avoid prolonged calorie counting (restrictive diets) day in and day out. You could choose to forego the potential short term weight loss to prevent long term health problems.

There's another problem with diets. Trending diets often neglect individuality and fail to consider the unique physiological and psychological needs of women. Women have different hormonal profiles compared to men, and their bodies respond differently to dietary interventions. Hormonal fluctuations during and after menopause can impact metabolism and fat storage. **Failing to address these hormonal nuances in diet plans can hinder sustainable fat loss efforts for women** (see hormone balancing, Chapter 2).

Dr. Fung, nephrologist and bestselling author of *The Obesity Code,* gave a lecture in 2016 on the way science shows we burn fuel.[17] Many people struggle to lose weight and keep it

---

[16] Oh TJ et al. Body-weight fluctuation and incident diabetes mellitus, cardiovascular disease and mortality: a 16-year prospective cohort study. *The Journal of Clinical Endocrinology & Metabolism.* 2018;104(3):639-646. doi:10.1210/jc.2018-01239

[17] Jason Fung. Fasting and Weight Loss - Solving the Two-Compartment problem. *YouTube.* Published online March 15, 2016. https://www.youtube.com/watch?v=ETkwZIi3R7w

off because they don't understand how the body stores energy for fuel. Your liver stores sugar as glycogen to burn as fuel after eating. You can think of that as your internal refrigerator. What yo-yo dieting weight regain proves is that **how much we eat is not the secret to weight loss. The secret is accessing the other way your body stores energy; burning our fat.** You can think of that fat burning system as your freezer. It's in the basement, inconvenient, but it's there because the fridge has a limited capacity.

One of the top ranked diets is The Biggest Loser diet. It decreases calories daily (calorie counting) and increases exercise daily. It's known as "eat less, move more." After 30 weeks of this strict, harsh approach, the average weight loss was over 100 lbs. However, many of The Biggest Losers have gone public saying they gained the weight back. Why? Science shows the reason for weight regain is slowed down metabolism.

A 2016 study in the journal *Obesity* followed 14 of The Biggest Losers over six years. It found weight regain and metabolic slowing in 100% of them. They gained back 90 lbs they lost in the following six years. Why? The average metabolic slowdown was over 600 calories per day![18] Their metabolism slowed down by week 6 of the diet, and continued slowing down through week 30. This means that calorie counting conditioned the body to burn less calories per day. In other words, **calorie counting trained the body to burn less calories and store fat better than**

---

[18] See RMR in Figures 2, 5 in Fothergill E, et al. Persistent metabolic adaptation 6 years after "The Biggest Loser" competition. *Obesity.* 2016;24(8):1612-1619. doi:10.1002/oby.21538

before the diet. That is why The Biggest Losers gained the weight back.

If you think about it, that makes sense. We're built to withstand repeated episodes of *no* food, not *less* food. When we were cavemen we did not eat three times a day. There was no abundant food supply. Like bears, lions, and other animals, humans did not eat multiple times a day. We survived, like other animals, starving for days at a time before eating (fast/famine cycles). Bears can hibernate for weeks at a time and they survive without food during the fasting state. Similarly, the human body evolved to survive by storing fat to burn for energy when there was no food available. If you eat too many hours a day, keeping insulin high, you cannot get into your freezer to burn fat.

The weight loss lie: Eat less and move more to lose weight (calorie counting)

In the Women's Health Initiative study in 2006, nearly 50000 postmenopausal women were cutting 360 calories daily for seven years. If that caused fat loss, they would have lost over 200 lbs, about 30 lbs per year. The weight loss result? Zero pounds lost over seven years. In fact, they lost about five pounds the first year, then gained it back while calorie counting the following years.[19]

Why calorie counting failed for nearly 50000 postmenopausal women

In 1991 an analysis of 29 calorie counting studies showed if you cut 10% of calories per day for five years, your

---

[19] Howard BV, et al. Low-Fat dietary pattern and weight change over 7 years. *JAMA.* 2006;295(1):39. doi:10.1001/jama.295.1.39

metabolism slows down 10% (RMR drops 10%).[20] In other words, **the body adapts to decreased daily calories by slowing metabolism so that you burn no fat and do not lose weight.** This point is reinforced in a 2004 study that showed calorie counting alone does not improve fat burning in 50 obese women over 50.[21] If you are calorie counting, your body just adapts by burning less calories. We've known since the nineties that calorie counting always fails for weight loss.

In other words, research proves if you empty your liver (your fridge) of stored sugar without affecting insulin, you cannot burn your stored fat because you cannot access your freezer. So **your body will just burn less sugar when it cannot burn fat for energy**.

This bad advice of eating less and moving more is based on a one compartment model of human energy storage, as if all incoming calories are stored in one place. Based on this false premise, if you put less in, you'll lose weight. Wait a minute. We know our sugar and fat are *not* stored in the same place. **This bad advice of eating less is given to overweight people who can't keep the weight off. Then when they fail we blame them, not the advice.** That's blaming the victim.

By the same logic of calorie counting, you could say smoking too much causes smoking so smoking less would help quit smoking. That doesn't work because it does not address the

[20] Prentice AM, et al. Physiological responses to slimming. *Proceedings of the Nutrition Society.* 1991;50(2):441-458. doi:10.1079/pns19910055
[21] You T., et al. Effects of hypocaloric diet and exercise training on inflammation and adipocyte lipolysis in obese postmenopausal women. *J. Clin. Endocrinol. Metab.* 2004;89(4):1739–1746. doi: 10.1210/jc.2003-031310.

root cause which is the reason they smoke. With an alcoholic, drinking less alcohol each day does not cure alcoholism. Similarly, eating less calories each day does not lose weight. Moreover, everyone knows cutting calories does not work. Doctors, dieticians, and people in general know it does not work.

In fact, doctors know weight gain is based on hormones, not calories. Any doctor prescribing insulin knows this from the DCCT study in 2001 where insulin caused massive weight gain over nine years for over 30% of patients.[22] So doctors know if they prescribe insulin, it can cause major weight gain. They know high insulin does not cause weight loss. When your insulin stays high through regular eating, the body is signaled to store fat. You need low insulin to signal the body to burn fat (see below).

Ever wonder why smokers stay thin? Nicotine causes weight loss by affecting hormones - it has no effect on calories. A 2011 study on over 5000 women showed that smoking over ten years yielded lower weight compared to non-smokers.[23] Nicotine affects the sympathetic hormones: it raises adrenaline and metabolic rate and lowers appetite. Everyone knows smoking is bad for you, so no one will recommend it for weight loss, but it works by affecting hormones.

So what's the secret to successful weight loss? If you ask a six-year-old how to lose weight they will tell you "don't eat."

──────────────────────

[22] See Figure 1 in White NH, et al; Diabetes Control and Complications Trial (DCCT). Beneficial effects of intensive therapy of diabetes during adolescence: outcomes after the conclusion of the Diabetes Control and Complications Trial (DCCT). J Pediatr. 2001 Dec;139(6):804-12. doi: 10.1067/mpd.2001.118887.
[23] Audrain-McGovern J, Benowitz NL. Cigarette smoking, nicotine, and body weight. Clin Pharmacol Ther. 2011 Jul;90(1):164-8. doi: 10.1038/clpt.2011.105.

Dr. Fung will tell you that's right. That's fasting. Yet this simple truth somehow escaped 99% of doctors and dieticians.

Another reason diets fail is they often lack a focus on behavior change and habits. Sustainable fat loss requires healthy lifestyle habits, including not overeating, eating healthy, regular physical activity, and stress management. **The reason habits are so effective for weight loss is they require no willpower.** Simply following a rigid diet for a short period without addressing underlying behaviors and habits is unlikely to yield long term success.

The main reason yo-yo dieting does not work is that it has no effect on insulin. Instead of relying on short-lived diet trends, a simpler, sustainable weight loss approach involves changing how many hours you eat each day (fasting). Counting the hours you eat is foolproof, unlike calorie counting, and it affects hormones that signal your body what to do with body fat.

Hormone changes after we eat

Our whole body runs on hormones, instructions on how much to pump blood, how much body heat to generate, etc. So ignoring the hormonal side of things is not a great idea... [Weight] is not just about calories in and calories out. When you eat, insulin goes up telling the body to store calories as body fat for later use. <u>What you cannot do when insulin is high is burn fat... if you cut calories the body can lower the</u>

metabolic rate to find balance and body fat stays the
same.[24]

- _Jason Fung, MD in a lecture on weight loss to other physicians in 2022: "Intermittent Fasting and Reversing Type 2 Diabetes"_

Before we discuss optimizing female hormones for lasting weight loss, we need to understand what our hormones do when we eat and when we don't. Dr. Cahill is credited as the father of fasting and he broke down fasting into five stages that have been somewhat refined since. For clarity, here is Dr. Cahill's original definition of the stages of fasting based on hormone levels in patients fasting for eight days.[25]

Stage 1: 0-4h after you last ate
Insulin goes up, all cells burn sugar as fuel. Insulin is one nutrient sensor that detects food to signal the body to store fat in fat cells (the other sensor detects protein, mTOR).

Stage 2: 4-16h after you last ate
Insulin falls, mTOR falls, adrenalin, cortisol, and growth hormone levels rise from the stress of not eating. These are called counter-regulatory hormones as they run counter to insulin. The body is digesting food. Most cells are using sugar for energy. Based on original research, for 16 hours after you last ate you are burning mostly sugar, not fat. Good

---

[24] Jason Fung. Science of Intermittent Fasting | Intermittent Fasting | Jason Fung. _YouTube_. Published online July 17, 2022. https://www.youtube.com/watch?v=6aiR1mFD7Gw at 16:35
[25] Cahill GF Jr, et al. 1966. Hormone-fuel interrelationships during fasting. J. Clin. Invest. 45:1751–69. See also Owen OE, et al. Liver and kidney metabolism during prolonged starvation. _Journal of Clinical Investigation._ 1969;48(3):574-583. doi:10.1172/jci106016

news! **Dr. Mattson co-authored a 2018 study stating fat burning starts 12 hours after you last ate.**[26] This means the more you fast over 12 hours, the more you burn fat.

Stage 3: 16-24h after you ate, aka **Autophagy**
mTOR spikes as glycogen reserves are depleted, the body makes glucose out of protein for fuel (see Autophagy in Chapter 2). This breaks down dysfunctional pieces of your cellular machinery and repairs and rejuvenates tissue. This way when you lose weight it does not yield loose skin.

Stage 4: 24h-48h+ after you ate, aka **Ketosis**
Since the brain can use only sugar for energy, the body changes your fat into ketones (i.e. burns fat). The ketones can enter the brain through the blood brain barrier. **The whole body is burning only fat 24 hours after you last ate.**

Stage 5: 6+ days extended fast, aka Protein Conservation
Hunger hormone ghrelin plummets because the whole body is running on only your body fat stores. This is why people can do 30- or 60-day fasts: they don't experience hunger at the extended fasting stage. Please note Stage 5 is beyond the scope of this book but it's included for reference.

You can see since insulin signals your body to store fat you have to lower insulin to burn fat. How do you lower insulin for fat burning and long term weight loss?

---

[26] Anton SD, et al. Flipping the metabolic switch: Understanding and applying the health benefits of fasting. *Obesity*. 2017;26(2):254-268. doi:10.1002/oby.22065

Long term weight loss

If you're in the habit of not eating after dinner it's not difficult [and] you have a weight loss habit that requires no willpower... The simplest rule of weight loss is just don't eat all the time. This is a very simple rule you can explain in 30 seconds that says don't eat between this hour and this hour.

- *Jason Fung, MD in lecture to other physicians on fasting and weight loss, May 11, 2022,[27] bestselling author of The Obesity Code*

Worldwide obesity prevalence has steadily increased over the last 40 years in Europe and America. Obesity is twice as prevalent in America compared to Europe (40% vs. 20%).[28] Obesity is a major risk factor for common diseases including coronary artery disease, type 2 diabetes, high blood pressure, and several types of cancer. All of these reduce both quality of life and lifespan.

The Study of Women's Health Across the Nation in the journal *Menopause* showed women gain fat during the menopause transition. Women gained roughly 14 lbs of fat from ten years before to about four years after menopause.[29]

---

[27] Jason Fung. Science of Intermittent Fasting | Intermittent Fasting | Jason Fung. *YouTube*. Published online July 17, 2022. https://www.youtube.com/watch?v=6aiR1mFD7Gw at 43:58 and 44:38
[28] Eglseer D, et al. Nutrition and Exercise Interventions to Improve Body Composition for Persons with Overweight or Obesity Near Retirement Age: A Systematic Review and Network Meta-Analysis of Randomized Controlled Trials. *Advances in Nutrition*. 2023;14(3):516-538. doi:10.1016/j.advnut.2023.04.001
[29] El Khoudary SR, et al. The menopause transition and women's health at midlife: a progress report from the Study of Women's Health Across the Nation (SWAN). Menopause. 2019 Oct;26(10):1213-1227. doi: 10.1097/GME.0000000000001424.

This is because research shows fat tends to be stored as abdominal fat after menopause due to lower hormone activity in the lower body.[30] So it's much harder to lose weight around menopause.

Before discussing the most effective method to lose fat, here are the criteria for "overweight" and "obese." Harvard will tell you the World Health Organization defines normal weight as body mass index (BMI) of 18.5 to 24.9.[31] If you measure above this, you are overweight: BMI of 25-30. Obesity is BMI over 30.

What do doctors advise for weight loss? A 2020 clinical practice guideline stated "decreased food intake and increased physical activity trigger a cascade of metabolic and hormonal mechanisms... effective tools in the long term management of obesity."[32] It follows that **patients would be advised to eat less and move more.** Yet everyone knows this does not work (as discussed above). What does science show always works for lasting weight loss?

The science of long term weight loss

A 2011 study on **107 overweight perimenopausal women reported 14 lbs lost over six months.[33] This**

---

[30] El-Zayat SR, Sibaii H, El-Shamy KA. Physiological process of fat loss. *Bulletin of the National Research Centre.* 2019;43(1). doi:10.1186/s42269-019-0238-z
[31] Body fat. The Nutrition Source. Published February 2, 2023. https://www.hsph.harvard.edu/nutritionsource/healthy-weight/measuring-fat/
[32] Wharton S, et al. Obesity in adults: a clinical practice guideline. *Canadian Medical Association Journal.* 2020;192(31):E875-E891. doi:10.1503/cmaj.191707
[33] Harvie, MN et al. The effects of intermittent or continuous energy restriction on weight loss and metabolic disease risk markers: a

11

was accomplished via intermittent fasting (IF).
Researchers concluded intermittent fasting "is effective in regards to weight loss… **a sustainable alternative for weight loss** and reducing disease risk."

Several studies show intermittent fasting facilitates weight loss and lowers body fat. A 2009 study on obese women demonstrated alternate-day fasting resulted in significant loss of body fat compared to calorie counting.[34] In this study 12 **obese women practiced alternate-day fasting for eight weeks. They lost 12.6 lbs in two months.** If you want to lose over 10 lbs, you could decide to fast every other day for two months, without changing what you eat and how you exercise.

A 2013 study showed alternate-day fasting yielded significant weight loss and reduced body fat compared to calorie counting.[35] This study involved **overweight perimenopausal women who ate every other day for 12 weeks. They lost 11.5 lbs in three months and 70% of it was fat.** If you want to lose fat, you could decide to eat every other day for three months.

A 2015 study testing three five day cycles of fasting-mimicking diet showed 3% weight loss, mostly abdominal

---

randomized trial in young overweight women. Int J Obes (Lond). 2011 May;35(5):714-27. doi: 10.1038/ijo.2010.171.
[34] Varady KA, et al. Short-term modified alternate-day fasting: a novel dietary strategy for weight loss and cardioprotection in obese adults. Am J Clin Nutr. 2009, 90: 1138-1143. 10.3945/ajcn.2009.28380.
[35] See Figure 2 in Varady KA, et al. Alternate day fasting for weight loss in normal weight and overweight subjects: a randomized controlled trial. *Nutrition Journal.* 2013;12(1). doi:10.1186/1475-2891-12-146

fat.[36] Not only does intermittent fasting burn fat, it can burn belly fat.

Still not convinced? **A 2017 review of 11 studies in the *Annual Review of Nutrition* found that IF was associated with a significant reduction in body weight and body fat.**[37] Additionally, the review found that IF was well-tolerated and did not lead to any side effects. Bonus effects included lower levels of disease risk factors. **This means you can lose fat and inches off your waist via intermittent fasting with no side effects.**

Moreover, a review of 40 studies showed 7-11 lbs lost within ten weeks of intermittent fasting. [38] Another study of 29 women up to 65 used alternate-day fasting. It showed **weight loss of 12 lbs in two months plus nearly three inches off the waist!**[39] If you want to lose weight and inches off your waist, you could eat every other day for two months.

Another review of 25 studies showed the most effective, sustainable method of losing inches off your waist involved the 5:2 fast.[40] It yielded 7% weight loss over 12 months. This

---

[36] Brandhorst S, et al. A Periodic Diet that Mimics Fasting Promotes Multi-System Regeneration, Enhanced Cognitive Performance, and Healthspan. *Cell metabolism*. 2015;22:86–99.

[37] See Table 2 in Patterson RE, Sears DD. Metabolic effects of intermittent fasting. *Annual Review of Nutrition*. 2017;37(1):371-393. doi:10.1146/annurev-nutr-071816-064634

[38] Seimon RV, et al. Do intermittent diets provide physiological benefits over continuous diets for weight loss? A systematic review of clinical trials. *Mol Cell Endocrinol*. 2015 Dec 15;418:153-72

[39] See Table 1 in Varady KA, et al. Effects of weight loss via high fat vs. low fat alternate day fasting diets on free fatty acid profiles. *Sci. Rep.* 2015;5:7561.

[40] Varady KA, et al. Cardiometabolic benefits of intermittent fasting. *Annual Review of Nutrition*. 2021;41(1):333-361. doi:10.1146/annurev-nutr-052020-041327

would be like a 200 lb woman staying 14 lbs lighter for a year. With 5:2 you eat normally five days a week plus 500 calories for two days. In other words, **fasting just two days a week is scientifically shown to be the most effective, sustainable way to lower waist size.**

By losing weight you also want to look leaner, right? In addition to weight loss, IF preserves lean muscle. A 2020 review of alternate-day fasting showed lean muscle preservation compared to calorie counting.[41] It was superior for weight loss and cholesterol with lower risk of weight regain. **This means it's healthier to eat every other day versus strict calorie counting every day!** If you want to be leaner you could fast every other day, which was already proven to lose 12 lbs in two months.

A 2023 review of 48 studies on lean muscle found that 5:2 intermittent fasting did not decrease muscle mass. It found **"the most effective strategy for loss of fat while maintaining or increasing muscle mass was the combination of energy restriction [fasting] and exercise."**[42] This means intermittent fasting does not burn muscle alongside regular exercise (see Introduction).

_____

[41] Park J, et al. Effect of alternate-day fasting on obesity and cardiometabolic risk: A systematic review and meta-analysis. *Metabolism.* 2020;111:154336. doi:10.1016/j.metabol.2020.154336. See also Figure 1 FFM in Heilbronn LK, et al. Alternate-day fasting in nonobese subjects: effects on body weight, body composition, and energy metabolism. *The American Journal of Clinical Nutrition.* 2005;81(1):69-73. doi:10.1093/ajcn/81.1.69

[42] See Figure 3B in Eglseer D, et al. Nutrition and Exercise Interventions to Improve Body Composition for Persons with Overweight or Obesity Near Retirement Age: A Systematic Review and Network Meta-Analysis of Randomized Controlled Trials. *Advances in Nutrition.* 2023;14(3):516-538. doi:10.1016/j.advnut.2023.04.001

By now you may be asking **if the science of IF for weight loss is indisputable, why didn't my medical doctor (MD) tell me about this?** As Dr. Fung said in a lecture to doctors about reversing diabetes, he did not know his patient did not need to be overweight and diabetic for 15 years.[43] MDs are trained to keep you alive with medication and surgery. If there's a nonmedicinal, nonsurgical approach that works, MDs are not trained to know it. Your MD cannot tell you what s/he does not know.

By burning fat, increasing metabolic rate, and preserving lean muscle, intermittent fasting offers significant benefits for women over 50. It is a proven method for women looking to lose weight and inches off their waist.

Please note it is important to approach IF after consulting a healthcare professional, especially if you have health conditions and take medication. To learn why fasting burns fat long term see Chapter 3. Continue to Chapter 2 to discover the myriad of health benefits from fasting for women after menopause.

---

[43] Swiss Re. Fasting can reverse type 2 diabetes by Jason Fung. *YouTube*. Published online October 20, 2023. https://www.youtube.com/watch?v=rg_vLxyQ9Ic at 2:30

Chapter 2

The Healing Power of Intermittent Fasting

Before discussing the fasting benefits for women's health, know that if you are sick you are not alone. The CDC stated in 2020 that 42% of adult women are obese and 45% have high blood pressure.[44] Looking after your family will be more difficult if you are sick. Research also shows 29% of women will develop Alzheimer's.[45] You are about to discover the incredible healing power of intermittent fasting.

Mental performance and brain health

Mental health issues are prevalent in perimenopausal women. Research shows 80–85% of all women experience unpleasant menopausal symptoms. The most common symptoms include hot flashes, irritability, mood swings, anxiety, and emotional instability.[46] Whether you are menopausal or postmenopausal, intermittent fasting (IF) supports mental function and brain health. Several studies have explored the effects of intermittent fasting on cognitive performance, mood, learning, and the prevention of Alzheimer's.

---

[44] FastStats. Womens Health.
https://www.cdc.gov/nchs/fastats/womens-health.htm
[45] Brookmeyer R, Abdalla N. Estimation of lifetime risks of Alzheimer's disease dementia using biomarkers for preclinical disease. Alzheimers Dement. 2018 Aug;14(8):981-988. doi: 10.1016/j.jalz.2018.03.005.
[46] Elavsky S, McAuley E. Physical activity and mental health outcomes during menopause: A randomized controlled trial. *Ann Behav Med.* 2007;33:132–42.

Before we dive in, did you know virtually all of our philosophical wisdom came from the ancient Greeks? Some of the greatest minds in history fasted for mental performance: Hippocrates, Plato, and Socrates. Hippocrates is credited as the first physician to prescribe fasting for healing.[47]

Consider how you feel after Christmas or Thanksgiving dinner. How mentally clear and focused do you feel after a giant meal? Most people feel brain fog and even fall asleep after such a big meal. How do you feel when you do *not* eat after the initial hunger passes? *More* focused.

Do you want to feel less moody, anxious, or irritable? A 2007 study showed fasting can reduce anxiety and depression and improve social functioning.[48] Women suffering mood swings, anxiety, or irritability will be happy to hear this: a 2013 review of clinical studies showed fasting improved mood, alertness, and provided a sense of peace.[49] If you want to feel at peace, less moody, anxious, and sad, you can fast.

Do you want to feel more focused and happy? Research shows fasting periods like fasting-mimicking diet can lead to

---

[47] Wang Y, Wu R. The effect of fasting on human metabolism and psychological health. *Disease Markers*. 2022;2022:1-7. doi:10.1155/2022/5653739
[48] Ghahremani M, Delshad Noghabi A, Tavakolizadeh J. Evaluating the effect of fasting on mental health. *J Gonabad Univ Med Sci Health Serv*. :1379–1
[49] Fond G, et al. Fasting in mood disorders: Neurobiology and effectiveness. A review of the literature. *Psychiatry Res*. 2013;209:253–8.

increased awareness, attention, mental acuity, and feelings of euphoria, reducing symptoms of depression.[50]

For a better understanding of fasting and mental performance, consider what fasting does to your hormones. When you fast you are under stress, releasing adrenaline during fight or flight mode. This instinctive response increases your focus and mental sharpness. The adrenaline response to fasting optimizes learning.[51] It also increases resistance to damage associated with dementia. Fasting raises stress hormone levels as insulin levels drop (counter-regulatory hormones). This helps your learning and memory. One 2009 study showed eating fewer daily calories boosts verbal memory.[52] It follows that IF improves memory, since restricting the time you have to eat could result in eating less each day.

In a three-year study of 99 seniors, IF improved mental performance by reducing inflammation and DNA damage.[53] The analysis showed that IF may improve mental functions via various pathways including ketone synthesis and glycolysis. **Adults who practiced IF regularly for three years enjoyed better cognitive scores and superior mental performance.**

---

[50] Salvadori G, Mirisola MG, Longo VD. Intermittent and periodic fasting, hormones, and cancer prevention. *Cancers*. 2021;13(18):4587. doi:10.3390/cancers13184587

[51] Fond G, et al. Fasting in mood disorders: Neurobiology and effectiveness. A review of the literature. *Psychiatry Res*. 2013;209:253–8.

[52] Witte AV, et al. Caloric restriction improves memory in elderly humans. Proc Natl Acad Sci U S A 2009; 106: 1255-60.39.

[53] Ooi TC, et al. Intermittent Fasting Enhanced the Cognitive Function in Older Adults with Mild Cognitive Impairment by Inducing Biochemical and Metabolic changes: A 3-Year Progressive Study. *Nutrients*. 2020;12(9):2644. doi:10.3390/nu12092644

Do you know anyone with Alzheimer's or dementia? Do you want to prevent it? Dr. Mattson authored a 2006 study describing how IF can prevent neuron damage and death.[54] Based on his research, alternating periods of sugar burning and fat burning via IF may increase cellular stress resistance and repair damaged proteins and cells. Ultimately, what do you want for peak mental performance (or youthful nerve function)? It's called autophagy.

Autophagy benefits

The 2016 Nobel Prize in Human Physiology was awarded to Dr. Ohsumi. His cutting edge research on autophagy mechanisms started a cascade of studies on activating it to prevent diseases like Alzheimer's. OK, what is autophagy?

This is the natural self-healing process of your cells to recycle usable parts and remove dysfunctional proteins and other parts. In 2019 a review in *The New England Journal of Medicine* explained this cellular repair and rejuvenation process:

> Autophagy enables cells to remove oxidatively damaged proteins and mitochondria and recycle undamaged molecular constituents while reducing protein synthesis to conserve energy and resources. These [cell repair] pathways are untapped or

---

[54] Martin B, Mattson MP, Maudsley S. Caloric restriction and intermittent fasting: Two potential diets for successful brain aging. *Ageing Research Reviews.* 2006;5(3):332-353. doi:10.1016/j.arr.2006.04.002

suppressed in persons who overeat and are sedentary.[55]

This means the more you eat and the less you move you will age faster, with declining mental performance.

If you think of remodeling a kitchen, before you can rebuild and make it look new, you have to rip out the old parts: the counters, cabinets, flooring, etc. In order to rebuild and rejuvenate your cells and tissues, you need autophagy to clear out the old, dysfunctional proteins and other parts, replacing them with rebuilt parts.

If you extend your daily fast beyond 16 hours it triggers autophagy. In this review, Dr. Mattson went on to say eating every other day can delay the onset and progression of Alzheimer's and Parkinson's. IF increases stress resistance of nerve cells via several mechanisms: autophagy, antioxidant defenses, boosting mitochondrial function, and DNA repair.[56] This could help prevent Alzheimer's, Parkinson's, Lou-Gehrig's disease (ALS) and other neurodegenerative diseases.[57]

Based on Dr. Mattson's review, if you know women eating over seven hours a day, they would NOT benefit from cell repair and rejuvenation of their tissues and organs. **Women who want to enjoy peak mental performance could repair and rejuvenate nerve tissue by eating all food**

[55] De Cabo R, Mattson MP. Effects of intermittent fasting on health, aging, and disease. *The New England Journal of Medicine.* 2019;381(26):2541-2551. doi:10.1056/nejmra1905136
[56] Menzies FM, et al. Autophagy and neurodegeneration: pathogenic mechanisms and therapeutic opportunities. Neuron 2017; 93: 1015-34
[57] Ibid

within seven hours a day, triggering autophagy. This is simply time-restricted feeding.

You may be able to trigger autophagy with a low protein diet as well since reducing protein intake signals the body there is no food (low protein intake reduces mTOR). This is one of several reasons why eating a low protein diet is recommended by Dr. Longo for a long, healthy life.[58]

IF also enhances GABA hormone activity which can prevent seizures and toxic effects on neurons causing dysfunction and death of nerve cells (excitotoxicity). [59] This is what causes dementia and Alzheimer's; it's what we want to avoid.

Do you know any women with MS? Two recent studies showed MS patients practicing IF improve symptoms within two months.[60,61] The 2018 study showed 36 MS patients following a 5:2 fasting regimen enjoyed significant improvement in emotional wellbeing and depression scores.

Research shows IF helps women after menopause: it enhances mood, learning, memory, and reduces anxiety and depression symptoms. It can also prevent diseases like Alzheimer's and improve MS symptoms. IF promotes brain health. One of the most powerful ways fasting improves your nerve cells is by activating autophagy. If you want to feel less

---

[58] For more on protein, see Chapter 1 in *The Whole Foods Diet for Longevity*
[59] Brocchi A, et al. Effects of intermittent fasting on brain metabolism. *Nutrients.* 2022;14(6):1275. doi:10.3390/nu14061275
[60] Choi IY, et al. A diet mimicking fasting promotes regeneration and reduces autoimmunity and multiple sclerosis symptoms. Cell Rep 2016; 15: 2136-46.
[61] Fitzgerald KC, et al. Effect of intermittent vs. daily calorie restriction on changes in weight and patient-reported outcomes in people with multiple sclerosis. Mult Scler Relat Disord 2018; 23: 33-9.

brain fog, mood swings, anxiety, or depression, you could eat all food in seven hours a day on a periodic basis. Autophagy could also help repair and rejuvenate skin and hair. It could be that it helps wrinkles and cellulite as much as nerve cells.

Balancing hormones

Some women are reluctant to start intermittent fasting (IF) because they believe there are side effects to sex hormone levels like estrogen and progesterone. A 2022 review of the effects of IF on sex hormone levels showed no change in estrogen and gonadotropin levels in women.[62] The only changes were decreased testosterone and increased beneficial protein levels in obese women before menopause. Decreased testosterone is good for women over 50 (see below). This indicates IF has no adverse effects on female hormones after menopause.

Estrogen

This is the main female reproductive hormone and is involved in the development and maintenance of female reproductive tissues and menstrual cycle.[63] This is why estrogen levels fall after menopause (i.e. no cycle). Estrogen can improve mood swings, night sweats, and vaginal symptoms of menopause, such as dryness, itching, burning, and discomfort with intercourse.[64] It can also help prevent bone loss and osteoporosis. Estrogen also reduces appetite,

---

[62] Cienfuegos S, Corapi S, Gabel K, et al. Effect of intermittent fasting on reproductive hormone levels in females and males: a review of human trials. *Nutrients*. 2022;14(11):2343. doi:10.3390/nu14112343
[63] Lizcano, F.; Guzmán, G. Estrogen deficiency and the origin of obesity during menopause. *BioMed Res. Int.* **2014**, *2014*, 757461.
[64] Professional CCM. Estrogen. Cleveland Clinic. https://my.clevelandclinic.org/health/body/22353-estrogen

opposite progesterone.[65] Women of all ages want optimal estrogen function.

Overweight women have higher levels of estrogens. A 2011 study showed these women have higher risk for breast cancer and polycystic ovarian syndrome (PCOS).[66] Weight loss interventions like IF have been shown to reduce estrogen levels in women with obesity down to optimal levels.[67] If you know an obese woman over 50, IF can improve her estrogen levels and lower her risk for breast cancer.

Do you know anyone with PCOS, the most common hormonal disease affecting women? One 2013 study measured time-restricted feeding and estrogen levels. It compared the effect of eating most food at dinner versus breakfast. Research shows that eating most of your calories later in the day can raise estrogen levels in women with PCOS.[68] Elevated testosterone is converted to estrogen in fat, leading to excess estrogen in women with obesity and PCOS.[69] Too much estrogen and testosterone are the primary

---

[65] Hirschberg AL. Sex hormones, appetite and eating behaviour in women. *Maturitas*. 2012;71(3):248-256.
doi:10.1016/j.maturitas.2011.12.016
[66] Campbell, K.L. et al. Reduced-calorie dietary weight loss, exercise, and sex hormones in postmenopausal women: Randomized controlled trial. *J. Clin. Oncol.* **2012**, *30*, 2314. See also Hormones, E. and Group, B.C.C. Circulating sex hormones and breast cancer risk factors in postmenopausal women: Reanalysis of 13 studies. *Br. J. Cancer* **2011**, *105*, 709.
[67] Stolzenberg-Solomon, R.Z. et al. Sex hormone changes during weight loss and maintenance in overweight and obese postmenopausal African-American and non-African-American women. *Breast Cancer Res.* **2012**, *14*, 3346–3356.
[68] See Table 1 in Jakubowicz, D. et al. Effects of caloric intake timing on insulin resistance and hyperandrogenism in lean women with polycystic ovary syndrome. *Clinical Science*. 2013;125(9):423-432.
doi:10.1042/cs20130071
[69] Ibid

causes of anovulation in PCOS.[70] Shifting the TRF eating window to early in the day may help women with obesity / PCOS to avoid further increases in estrogen.

Since IF optimizes estrogen in overweight women, a woman could use IF to reduce mood swings, night sweats, and vaginal symptoms: dryness, itching, burning, and discomfort with intercourse. It can also help prevent bone loss and osteoporosis with an added bonus of keeping weight off by reducing appetite.

Testosterone

Postmenopausal women with excess testosterone can grow excessive hair and develop scaly patches on their body and scalp.[71] **Studies show excess testosterone promotes insulin resistance in women.**[72] So **with excess testosterone you cannot burn fat.** In women with PCOS and obesity, weight loss has been shown to optimize testosterone and SHBG levels (i.e. decrease testosterone available by increasing SHBG).[73]

A study in 2021 was done on obese women with PCOS eating all food from 8am to 4pm (16:8) for five weeks. Eating all

---

[70] Cienfuegos S, et al. Effect of intermittent fasting on reproductive hormone levels in females and males: a review of human trials. *Nutrients*. 2022;14(11):2343. doi:10.3390/nu14112343

[71] Rosenfield, R.L. Hirsutism: Implications, etiology, and management. *American Journal of Obstetrics and Gynecology*. 1981;140(7):815-830. doi:10.1016/0002-9378(81)90746-8

[72] Diamond, M.P. et al. Effects of methyltestosterone on insulin secretion and sensitivity in women. *J. Clin. Endocrinol. Metab.* **1998**, *83*, 4420–4425.

[73] Pasquali, R. Obesity and androgens: Facts and perspectives. *Fertil. Steril.* **2006**, *85*, 1319–1340.

food in eight hours earlier in the day in just five weeks decreased total testosterone and body weight.[74] The decreased testosterone from IF lowered insulin and weight.

Another study looked at PCOS patients eating over half their food at breakfast versus dinner. The results showed testosterone-like androgens decreased significantly in the breakfast group relative to the dinner group.[75] Any side effects? None, but here were the bonus effects of fasting after 4pm: decreased body weight, inflammation, and insulin resistance. This research suggests fasting can significantly decrease testosterone in women with no cycle, especially if they eat all food before 4pm.

Sex hormone-binding globulin (SHBG)

This protein moves testosterone and estrogen to target tissues. The availability of your sex hormones is influenced by SHBG levels. More SHBG reduces available testosterone which benefits women. **Weight loss via IF has been shown to increase SHBG and improve insulin sensitivity in women with obesity** and PCOS.[76]

One 2011 study on obese women showed 5:2 fasting significantly increased SHBG. It also showed 7% weight loss after six months.[77] By binding testosterone, these women

74 Li, C. et al. Eight-hour time-restricted feeding improves endocrine and metabolic profiles in women with anovulatory polycystic ovary syndrome. *J. Transl. Med.* **2021**, *19*, 148.

75 Jakubowicz, D. et al. Effects of caloric intake timing on insulin resistance and hyperandrogenism in lean women with polycystic ovary syndrome. *Clin. Sci.* **2013**, *125*, 423–432.

76 Pugeat, M. et al.. Pathophysiology of sex hormone binding globulin (SHBG): Relation to insulin. *J. Steroid Biochem. Mol. Biol.* **1991**, *40*, 841–849.

77 Harvie, M.N. et al. The effects of intermittent or continuous energy restriction on weight loss and metabolic disease risk markers: A

had less free testosterone (and less insulin). That's good for weight loss. Similar increases were measured in five weeks of 16:8 fasting in women with PCOS.[78] This is especially true when all food is consumed before 4pm (i.e. eating from 8am to 4pm).

Progesterone

Progesterone has neuroprotective and bone preservation functions.[79] It could help you stay calm and is anti-osteoporosis. A two month time-restricted feeding study in 2022 showed no decrease in progesterone. This means IF does not lower your feeling of calm and does not increase unwanted symptoms like irritability, anxiety, mood swings or depression common in perimenopausal women. It also indicates IF can help prevent bone loss.

Insulin Sensitivity

There is significant research on insulin resistance associated with menopause. One 2011 study involving 61 perimenopausal, overweight women measured effects of intermittent fasting on insulin sensitivity.[80] Three months on a 5:2 IF regimen showed significant improvements in insulin

randomized trial in young overweight women. *Int. J. Obes.* **2011**, *35*, 714–727.

[78] Li, C. et al. Eight-hour time-restricted feeding improves endocrine and metabolic profiles in women with anovulatory polycystic ovary syndrome. *J. Transl. Med.* **2021**, *19*, 148.

[79] Graham JD, Clarke CL. Physiological action of progesterone in target tissues*. *Endocrine Reviews*. 1997;18(4):502-519. doi:10.1210/edrv.18.4.0308

[80] Harvie, M. et al. (2011). The effect of intermittent energy and carbohydrate restriction v. daily energy restriction on weight loss and metabolic disease risk markers in overweight women. British Journal of Nutrition, 105(3), 583-587.

sensitivity, suggesting that intermittent fasting can regulate insulin. This lessens the insulin resistance associated with menopause to promote weight loss.

A 2018 review investigated the effects of time-restricted feeding on insulin sensitivity. The participants followed a 16:8 time-restricted feeding window for ten weeks. The results revealed significant improvements in insulin sensitivity, blood pressure, and oxidative stress.[81] Research shows intermittent fasting can optimize insulin levels and metabolic health. In fact, research shows IF can optimize all of your hormones, including estrogen, testosterone, and progesterone.

Gut health

Studies have shown that alterations in the gut microbiome can significantly improve sex hormones and metabolism. **This means improving an abnormal gut microbiome can improve your health after menopause.**[82] **Clinical studies show intermittent fasting can improve the makeup and diversity of the gut microbes.** A 2021 study on periodic fasting (FMD) was shown to reduce gut permeability, buildup of toxins and systemic inflammation elevated in obesity.[83] That makes sense since we all know fasting has been a detox or cleanse for thousands of years.

---

[81] Barnosky, A. R. et al (2018). Intermittent fasting vs daily calorie restriction for type 2 diabetes prevention: a review of human findings. Translational Research, 164(4), 302-311. doi:10.1016/j.trsl.2014.05.013
[82] Qi, X. et al. The impact of the gut microbiota on the reproductive and metabolic endocrine system. *Gut Microbes* **2021**, *13*, 1894070.
[83] Mohr, A.E. et al. Recent advances and health implications of dietary fasting regimens on the gut microbiome. *Am. J. Physiol. Gastrointest. Liver Physiol.* **2021**, *320*, G847–G863.

In 2020 the *British Journal of Nutrition* found fasting helps various members of the gastrointestinal flora yielding byproducts helping our metabolism (butyrate, acetate, and mucin stimulants).[84] In other words, IF may optimize hormones by benefiting our gut health.

In addition to improving gut health with time-restricted feeding and fasting-mimicking diet, you can improve your microbiome with food. If you stop eating meat (rich in antibiotics) you stop reducing beneficial gut bacteria and benefit from their byproduct, resveratrol. This good gut bacteria helps maintain good estrogen and break down harmful estrogen.[85]

Cancer prevention

The pursuit of anti-aging and longevity is commonplace for women over 50. The second most common cause of death is cancer, according to the CDC, and nearly 40% of women will have cancer. [86] Intermittent fasting (IF) is shown to reduce risk of hormone-related and other cancers. This is one of several ways fasting promotes longevity.

---

[84] Zeb, F. et al. Effect of time-restricted feeding on metabolic risk and circadian rhythm associated with gut microbiome in healthy males. *Br. J. Nutr.* **2020**, *123*, 1216–1226.

[85] Qasem RJ. The estrogenic activity of resveratrol: a comprehensive review of *in vitro* and *in vivo* evidence and the potential for endocrine disruption. Crit Rev Toxicol. 2020 May;50(5):439-462. doi: 10.1080/10408444.2020.

[86] Lifetime risk of developing or dying from cancer. American Cancer Society. https://www.cancer.org/cancer/risk-prevention/understanding-cancer-risk/lifetime-probability-of-developing-or-dying-from-cancer.html

Breast Cancer

Excess fat affects circulating hormones, particularly in postmenopausal women, and can up your risk for breast cancer. In the Nurses Health Study over 49,000 postmenopausal women were followed for up to 24 years. The data suggested that weight gain during adult life, especially after menopause, increases the risk of breast cancer.[87] The Nurses Health Study found **weight loss after menopause is associated with a decreased risk of breast cancer.** Since IF is proven to lose weight, IF reduces your risk of breast cancer.

The Iowa Women's Health Study followed over 41,000 women over 15 years. The average weight gain from 18 to 50 was 24 lbs. The study showed weight gain after age 30 years was worse than weight gain before 30.[88] Data suggest prevention of weight gain between 18 years and menopause or weight loss and maintenance during these years reduces risk of breast cancer. Weight maintenance via IF would be a good choice for women who want to prevent breast cancer.

Furthermore, a 2021 clinical study in *The British Journal of Cancer* examined the effects of IF on 169 women with breast cancer.[89] The intervention involved two consecutive days of very low-calorie intake per week (FMD of 650-1000

---

[87] AH Eliassen, et al. Adult weight change and risk of postmenopausal breast cancer JAMA, 296 (2006), pp. 193-201

[88] Harvie M, et al. Association of Gain and Loss of Weight before and after Menopause with Risk of Postmenopausal Breast Cancer in the Iowa Women's Health Study. *Cancer Epidemiology, Biomarkers & Prevention.* 2005;14(3):656-661. doi:10.1158/1055-9965.epi-04-0001

[89] Harvie M, et al. Randomised controlled trial of intermittent vs continuous energy restriction during chemotherapy for early breast cancer. *British Journal of Cancer.* 2021;126(8):1157-1167. doi:10.1038/s41416-021-01650-0

calories). They found reduced IGF-1 and IGF-2 and adiponectin, indicating intermittent fasting can lower breast cancer risk. This study also found 100% of the fasting group receiving chemotherapy responded better than the calorie counting group. If you know anyone with early breast cancer, fasting-mimicking diet is proven helpful.

Moreover, a 2016 study on over 2400 breast cancer patients, 78% of whom were postmenopausal, found IF reduces breast cancer recurrence by 64%.[90] Let me repeat that for emphasis: **intermittent fasting reduces risk of breast cancer recurrence.** Fasting less than 13 hours per night (eating three meals a day) was associated with 36% increased risk of recurrence. These women fasted 13h per night for seven years. Were there side effects from seven years of IF? None. Bonus effects included decreased blood sugar and longer sleep for every additional two hours of fasting. This means breast cancer survivors eating in ten hours or less per day (practicing 14:10 TRF) have a 64% reduced risk of cancer recurrence, with more sleep and lower blood sugar as a bonus!

Ovarian Cancer

The five-year survival rate of ovarian cancer is 45%. It is the most lethal gynecological cancer. Animal studies show IF boosted anti-tumor immunity via natural killer T cell response.[91] This means IF activates your immune cells to naturally attack the ovarian cancer cells. This led to

---

[90] Marinac CR, et al. Prolonged nightly fasting and breast cancer prognosis. *JAMA Oncology*. 2016;2(8):1049. doi:10.1001/jamaoncol.2016.0164

[91] Udumula MP, et al. Abstract 2161: Fasting fueled ketogenesis inhibits ovarian cancer and promotes anti-tumor T cell response. *Cancer Research*. 2022;82(12_Supplement):2161. doi:10.1158/1538-7445.am2022-2161

improved survival rate. This suggests IF can restrict tumor growth and improve survival alone or in combination with immunotherapy. Human clinical studies will be forthcoming.

Endometrial Cancer

A world-class study on endometrial cancer in 1500 women is underway at the University of North Carolina. Endometrial cancer, which mainly affects postmenopausal women, is the most prevalent gynecologic cancer among American women, and rising.[92] By 2040, endometrial cancer is expected to displace colon cancer as the third most common cancer among women and the fourth leading cause of cancer death in women. So far in this study, "intermittent fasting appears far superior to other interventions like low or high fat diet and bariatric surgery."

Other Cancers

Preclinical studies and clinical trials have shown that intermittent fasting has anti-cancer benefits. Dr. Mattson has been researching fasting for over 20 years. He co-authored a 2019 review in *The New England Journal of Medicine.* He wrote that eating six hours per day

> is thought to impair energy metabolism in cancer cells inhibiting their growth... and may provide protection against cancer while bolstering the stress resistance of

---

[92] Well BLW. Lineberger leads endometrial cancer moonshot | UNC-Chapel Hill. The University of North Carolina at Chapel Hill. Published June 6, 2023. https://www.unc.edu/discover/lineberger-leads-endometrial-cancer-moonshot/#:~:text=Another%20study%20looks%20at%20the,diet%20and%20even%20bariatric%20surgery

normal cells... Several case studies involving patients with glioblastoma suggest that intermittent fasting can suppress tumor growth and extend survival.[93]

Dr. Mattson is saying that fasting strengthens healthy cells and weakens cancer cells. He's also saying fasting helps treat brain cancer. Since fasting "protects against cancer" while strengthening normal cells, fasting can prevent cancer.

Which other cancers can be prevented and treated with fasting? A 2004 review in the preeminent journal *Lancet* showed reduced IGF-1 from fasting can prevent colon and breast cancer.[94] Mutations in the human IGF-1R were found to protect against cancer and other diseases associated with aging. A 2008 study reported that most people living over 100 have this desirable mutation lowering IGF-1.[95] If you want to live over 100 you can do so preventing breast and colon cancer with IF.

Research in 2021 showed the fasting-mimicking diet is the most viable strategy for cancer prevention with no side effects, unlike other fasting methods or calorie counting, for four reasons.[96] First, it causes the most extreme drops in IGF-1, insulin, and leptin which facilitates anticancer effects.

---

[93] De Cabo R, Mattson MP. Effects of intermittent fasting on health, aging, and disease. *The New England Journal of Medicine*. 2019;381(26):2541-2551. doi:10.1056/nejmra1905136

[94] Renehan A.G., et al. Insulin-like growth factor (IGF)-I, IGF binding protein-3, and cancer risk: Systematic review and meta-regression analysis. *Lancet*. 2004;363:1346–1353. doi: 10.1016/S0140-6736(04)16044-3.

[95] Suh Y., et al. Functionally significant insulin-like growth factor I receptor mutations in centenarians. *Proc. Natl. Acad. Sci. USA*. 2008;105:3438–3442. doi: 10.1073/pnas.0705467105.

[96] Salvadori G, Mirisola MG, Longo VD. Intermittent and periodic fasting, hormones, and cancer prevention. *Cancers*. 2021;13(18):4587. doi:10.3390/cancers13184587

Second, FMD stimulates anticancer immunity. Third, it prevents muscle loss. Lastly, it can be combined with standard cancer treatments but also cancer prevention because it is sustainable for even frail, elderly people. If you know any women that don't get around much anymore, FMD is possible as it is only conducted for several days a month, preserves muscle, and does not require diet changes during eating windows. In fact, it's shown to be tolerated in hospital beds.

In a 2017 study the FMD group achieved an 11% drop in blood sugar and a 24% drop in IGF-1, remaining 15% lower than baseline levels after refeeding![97] This was done with five days of FMD cycles over three months. The FMD-dependent reduction in blood glucose and IGF-1 levels is anti-cancer.[98] Three FMD cycles also reduced CRP, an inflammatory marker in those at risk for diseases of aging. This means FMD is both anti-inflammatory and anti-cancer.

Researchers wrote periodic fasting via cycles of FMD could prevent obesity, inflammatory diseases and cancer.[99] Any FMD side effects? No. FMD bonuses included decreased blood pressure and lower weight and waist size, with a 3% loss in fat. The only increase was lean body mass, suggesting that it causes only fat loss.

---

[97] Wei M., et al. Fasting-mimicking diet and markers/risk factors for aging, diabetes, cancer, and cardiovascular disease. *Sci. Transl. Med.* 2017;9 doi: 10.1126/scitranslmed.aai8700.

[98] Stocks T., et al. Blood glucose and risk of incident and fatal cancer in the metabolic syndrome and cancer project (me-can): Analysis of six prospective cohorts. *PLoS Med.* 2009;6:e1000201. doi: 10.1371/journal.pmed.1000201.

[99] Wei M., et al. Fasting-mimicking diet and markers/risk factors for aging, diabetes, cancer, and cardiovascular disease. *Sci. Transl. Med.* 2017;9 doi: 10.1126/scitranslmed.aai8700.

FMD can also promote immune system regeneration and rejuvenation important for cancer development.[100] By boosting immunity cancer improves. This is because regenerative medicine is showing the most effective cancer treatment is immunotherapy; using your own immune cells to attack previously "incurable" cancers.[101] Better yet, FMD is effective when performed a few times a year in five day cycles! For this reason Dr. Longo, in good health, practices FMD twice a year for anti-cancer and longevity benefits.[102]

Research also shows fasting can be a treatment for cancer. A 2021 study found IF has immediate and long term effects on hormones including IGF-1, insulin, and leptin. In 2021 Dr. Longo wrote periodic fasting with FMD can reduce tumor incidence by reducing IGF-1, delaying aging, preventing DNA damage, and killing precancerous and cancer cells.[103] Again, research shows fasting can kill cancer cells.

In cancer progression fatty tissue exhibits increased leptin production with effects on insulin sensitivity, inflammation, cell proliferation and cell death.[104] Intermittent fasting reduces leptin by 40%, which inhibits cancer progression.[105]

---

[100] Brandhorst S., et al. A Periodic Diet that Mimics Fasting Promotes Multi-System Regeneration, Enhanced Cognitive Performance, and Healthspan. *Cell Metab.* 2015;22:86–99. doi: 10.1016/j.cmet.2015.05.012.

[101] For more on the emerging specialty of cancer immunotherapy, see Chapter 19 in Robbins T, Diamandis PH. *Life Force: How New Breakthroughs in Precision Medicine Can Transform the Quality of Your Life & Those You Love.* Simon and Schuster; 2022. pg 431 - 462

[102] Ibid

[103] Salvadori G, Mirisola MG, Longo VD. Intermittent and periodic fasting, hormones, and cancer prevention. *Cancers.* 2021;13(18):4587. doi:10.3390/cancers13184587

[104] Hursting SD, et al. Obesity, energy balance, and Cancer: New opportunities for Prevention. *Cancer Prevention Research.* 2012;5(11):1260-1272. doi:10.1158/1940-6207.capr-12-0140

[105] Ibid

Since leptin signals you to stop eating, this makes sense. If you feel less full with less leptin, this also signals the cancer cells there are less nutrients coming. This could lower cancer cell proliferation.

Does IF lower overall cancer risk?

In a 2009 analysis of over 275000 women, researchers wrote "abnormal glucose metabolism independent of [weight] is associated with an increased risk of cancer overall... with stronger associations among women."[106] The ten-year study found the higher the blood sugar, the higher the risk of getting and dying from cancer. It showed abnormal metabolism increases overall cancer risk, with significant increased risk in women for stomach, bladder, pancreatic, and uterine cancer. IF reduces overall cancer risk by improving glucose metabolism.

A 2008 **review of 141 studies in the preeminent journal *Lancet* showed weight loss is likely to reduce your risk of thirteen cancers linked to obesity!**[107] Since IF is associated with weight loss, your risk for these cancers drops with IF: breast, colon, kidney, esophageal, and thyroid. If you want to lower your risk for two of the top three lethal cancers in women, breast and colon cancer, intermittent fasting is a proven method. It also lowers your risk for 11 other cancers by losing weight.

---

[106] Stocks T, et al. Blood glucose and risk of incident and fatal cancer in the Metabolic Syndrome and Cancer Project (ME-CAN): Analysis of six prospective cohorts. *PLOS Medicine*. 2009;6(12):e1000201. doi:10.1371/journal.pmed.1000201

[107] Renehan AG, et al. Body-mass index and incidence of cancer: a systematic review and meta-analysis of prospective observational studies. *Lancet*. 2008;371:569–578. doi:10.1016/s0140-6736(08)60269-x

Inflammatory biomarker levels associated with cancer drop with IF about 2% for every 1% weight loss (CRP, TNF-α and IL-6).[108] These proteins are elevated with inflammation in obesity. TNF-α is associated with colon, liver, and skin cancer.[109] IL-6 is associated with colon cancer and lymphoma. **These data show IF is anti-inflammatory and significantly reduces most cancer risk biomarkers.**

A 2011 study showed the fasting-mimicking diet (FMD) lowered IGF-1 and the marker of inflammation in the blood (CRP) which are associated with cancer. Since the FMD variant of IF lowers cancer risk, you could choose to incorporate periods of FMD.[110] This is easier to maintain than alternate-day fasting (see Chapter 5).

If you want to lower your risk of two of the three most lethal cancers in women, breast and colon cancer, you could decide to incorporate IF into your lifestyle. Since fasting causes weight loss it lowers risk for 11 other types of cancer, and cellular pathways induced by fasting are anti-cancer overall.

By optimizing sex hormones, nerve function, and reducing the risk of dementia and cancer, intermittent fasting offers benefits for all women seeking to achieve hormonal balance, reduce postmenopausal symptoms, and live longer. You can

---

[108] Byers T, Sedjo RL. Does intentional weight loss reduce cancer risk? *Diabetes, Obesity and Metabolism.* 2011;13(12):1063-1072. doi:10.1111/j.1463-1326.2011.01464.x
[109] Harvey AE, Lashinger LM, Hursting SD. The growing challenge of obesity and cancer: an inflammatory issue. *Annals of the New York Academy of Sciences.* 2011;1229(1):45-52. doi:10.1111/j.1749-6632.2011.06096.x.
[110] J. Guevara-Aguirre, et al. Growth hormone receptor deficiency is associated with a major reduction in pro-aging signaling, cancer, and diabetes in humans. *Sci. Transl. Med.* **3**, 70ra13 (2011)

live longer fasting as it lowers cancer risk. What about lowering risk for the top cause of death?

Cardiovascular disease and anti-aging

Before discussing risk factors for heart disease, let's look at longevity at the cellular level. Dr. Longo is the Director of The Longevity Institute at USC, a leader in research on aging and age-related disease. His mission is to "help people live to 110 in good health."[111] His 40 years of research has shown anti-aging and longevity benefits.

Dr. Longo co-authored a 2017 study reporting the effects of intermittent fasting on cellular processes associated with aging. The study involved 50 participants who fasted 16 hours per day, three days per week, for three months.[112] Dr. Longo showed intermittent fasting activates cellular stress response pathways to enhance cellular repair and protect against age-related damage. In other words, **this study showed IF slows the aging process at a cellular level**. Furthermore, there were improvements in mitochondrial function, with an increase in oxidative capacity. This means you feel energized by fasting. By enhancing energy output and reducing free radicals, intermittent fasting can reduce oxidative stress to preserve cellular integrity and promote longevity.

---

[111] Robbins T, Diamandis PH. Life Force: How New Breakthroughs in Precision Medicine Can Transform the Quality of Your Life & Those You Love. Simon and Schuster; 2022. pg 285
[112] Mattson MP, Longo VD, Harvie M. Impact of intermittent fasting on health and disease processes. Ageing Res Rev. 2017 Oct;39:46-58. doi: 10.1016/j.arr.2016.10.005.

Live longer with people you love by intermittent fasting

Here is how Dr. Longo says you can live longer eating less food:

> The metabolic shift to ketone use and adaptations of the brain and nervous system to food deprivation play major roles in the disease-allaying effects of intermittent fasting.[113]

How does fasting increase lifespan? The leading cause of death is heart disease, per the World Health Organization, and risk factors include obesity, diabetes, high blood pressure, and high cholesterol. Do you know any women suffering one of these diseases? Intermittent fasting (IF) is proven for weight loss and reducing these diseases.

Reversing diabetes type 2

There is evidence to suggest that the fasting approach, where meals are restricted to an eight to 10-hour period of the daytime, is effective [for diabetics].[114]

- *Dr. Deb Wexler, Director of the Massachusetts General Diabetes Center, professor at Harvard Medical School*

---

[113] Ibid
[114] Harvard Health. Intermittent fasting: The positive news continues. Harvard Health. Published February 28, 2021. https://www.health.harvard.edu/blog/intermittent-fasting-surprising-update-2018062914156

Dr. Fung shared a four-month case study of one of his diabetic patients in a lecture to other physicians. For 11 years his patient was on metformin and insulin. He started eating one meal a day three days a week. In one month he was taken off insulin as his HbA1c dropped from 7.8 to 7.2.[115] He was cured in a few months: HbA1c dropped to 5.9. He reversed diabetes with IF and no refined carbs. **He got off meds in two months of IF after taking insulin for over ten years!**

Dr. Fung said in lecture that he failed this patient for 15 years. Remember, Dr. Fung is not just an MD; he's a nephrologist. In this lecture to other MDs, he astutely observed that MDs are not trained to prescribe fasting to reverse Type 2 diabetes. **He stressed that he can make anyone fat by giving them insulin**: "every patient of mine tells me they get fat [on insulin]. I give insulin, they get fat."[116] Fasting is the way you drop insulin to burn your stored sugar and fat, so blood sugar drops.

Is this an isolated diabetic success with fasting? Not at all. In fact, all versions of IF induce beneficial metabolic changes including normal blood sugar and the metabolic switch to burning fat (ketones).[117] A 2019 study of 31 women with Type 2 diabetes found that three months eating nine hours per day dropped HbA1c 1.4%. **That's a significant improvement in blood sugar via IF without changes in meds.** These

---

[115] Ku M, Ramos M, Fung J. Therapeutic fasting as a potential effective treatment for type 2 diabetes: A 4-month case study. *Journal of Insulin Resistance.* 2017;1(1). doi:10.4102/jir.v2i1.31
[116] Swiss Re. Fasting can reverse type 2 diabetes by Jason Fung. *YouTube.* Published online October 20, 2023.
https://www.youtube.com/watch?v=rg_vLxyQ9Ic at 10:50
[117] Ku M, Ramos M, Fung J. Therapeutic fasting as a potential effective treatment for type 2 diabetes: A 4-month case study. *Journal of Insulin Resistance.* 2017;1(1). doi:10.4102/jir.v2i1.31

women also lost almost two inches off their waist size in three months.[118]

We've known fasting reverses diabetes for over 20 years. A 1998 study in the journal *Diabetes Care* showed normalized HbA1c by adding periodic fasting; fasting for five days per week every five weeks over 15 weeks.[119] If you know a diabetic she could fast for five day periods every five weeks just three times to get off medication.

Dr. Fung co-authored a 2018 study where 4:3 intermittent fasting (eating one meal a day three times a week) reversed insulin resistance in type 2 diabetics.[120] Moreover, research in *The New England Journal of Medicine* revealed some patients on six hour TRF regimens and doctor supervision were able to reverse Type 2 diabetes and be taken off insulin.[121]

A 2022 study in a journal of clinical endocrinology showed IF cured 47% of diabetics.[122] Their diabetes was reversed in three months fasting and stayed in remission for six months.

---

[118] Kesztyüs D, et al. Adherence to Time-Restricted Feeding and Impact on abdominal obesity in primary care patients: Results of a pilot study in a Pre–Post design. *Nutrients*. 2019;11(12):2854. doi:10.3390/nu11122854

[119] Williams KV, et al. The effect of short periods of caloric restriction on weight loss and glycemic control in type 2 diabetes. *Diabetes Care*. 1998;21:2–8.

[120] Furmli S, et al. Therapeutic use of intermittent fasting for people with type 2 diabetes as an alternative to insulin. BMJ Case Rep 2018; 2018:bcr-2017-221854.

[121] De Cabo R, Mattson MP. Effects of intermittent fasting on health, aging, and disease. *The New England Journal of Medicine*. 2019;381(26):2541-2551. doi:10.1056/nejmra1905136

[122] Yang X, et al. Effect of an intermittent calorie-restricted diet on Type 2 diabetes remission: a randomized controlled trial. *The Journal of Clinical Endocrinology & Metabolism*. 2022;108(6):1415-1424. doi:10.1210/clinem/dgac661

The remission rate was only 2.8% for diabetics eating as usual. In other words, **research shows nearly half of type 2 diabetics can be cured by fasting within three months**. Eating more than three times a day they stay on meds.

Let's stop and think about this. You can enter and sustain the fat burning state AND lower blood sugar to cure diabetes using IF. **You don't have to change what you eat or how much you eat to enjoy lower weight and blood sugar, just when you eat.**

You can see IF can prevent and reverse Type 2 diabetes. In fact, Dr. Longo wrote metformin has been shown to be anti-aging via the same pathways that lower oxidative stress and DNA damage activated by IF.[123] You can get these anti-aging drug benefits without the metformin.

Lower blood pressure and cholesterol

Does IF also lower blood pressure? Yes. A 2018 study in the journal *Nutrition and Healthy Aging* showed those doing time-restricted feeding (16:8) had lower systolic blood pressure in three months (7 units lower).[124] They also enjoyed a 0.5% decrease in their visceral fat, which is linked to an increased risk of chronic diseases. These were bonus effects from fasting, on top of lower blood pressure!

---

[123] Longo VD, Panda S. Fasting, circadian rhythms, and Time-Restricted feeding in healthy lifespan. *Cell Metabolism.* 2016;23(6):1048-1059. doi:10.1016/j.cmet.2016.06.001

[124] Gabel K, et al. Effects of 8-hour time restricted feeding on body weight and metabolic disease risk factors in obese adults: A pilot study. *Nutrition and Healthy Aging.* 2018;4(4):345-353. doi:10.3233/nha-170036

A 2016 study found that IF dropped systolic blood pressure 13 units. The study found that IF improved endothelial function and lowered blood pressure by increasing the production of nitric oxide, a molecule that helps dilate blood vessels.[125] Endothelial dysfunction is an early marker of atherosclerosis, which is a leading cause of heart disease.

Does IF also lower cholesterol? Yes. Reviews of alternate-day fasting studies show fat loss of 3-12 lbs and total cholesterol dropping up to 21%.[126] In one study 29 women ate every other day for two months reducing LDL cholesterol 24%.[127]

A 2012 *Nutrition Journal* study examined the effects of alternate-day fasting on cardiovascular risk factors in overweight women.[128] The women followed alternate-day fasting for eight weeks. The results showed significant reductions in body weight, total cholesterol, triglycerides, and blood pressure. These findings suggest that alternate-day fasting is an effective treatment for overweight women that also lowers heart disease risk.

In a 2007 study, nine obese people eating every other day lowered cholesterol by 9.3 units. They also lost 8% of their

[125] Esmaeilzadeh F, Van De Borne P. Does intermittent fasting improve microvascular endothelial function in healthy middle-aged subjects? *Biology and Medicine*. 2016;8(6). doi:10.4172/0974-8369.1000337

[126] Tinsley GM, La Bounty PM. Effects of intermittent fasting on body composition and clinical health markers in humans. *Nutr. Rev.* 2015;73:661–674.

[127] See Table 1 in Varady KA, et al. Effects of weight loss via high fat vs. low fat alternate day fasting diets on free fatty acid profiles. *Scientific Reports*. 2015;5(1). doi:10.1038/srep07561

[128] Klempel MC, et al. Intermittent fasting combined with calorie restriction is effective for weight loss and cardio-protection in obese women. *Nutrition Journal*. 2012;11(1). doi:10.1186/1475-2891-11-98

starting weight in eight weeks.[129] This would be like **a 170 lb woman lowering cholesterol and losing 13 lbs in just two months** without changing what she eats or her workouts! The study also found striking reductions in markers of oxidative stress and inflammation.

Dr. Ornish spent 40 years researching nutrition and concluded "the vast majority of common diseases are caused by oxidative stress and inflammation."[130] If you want to live disease free, alternate-day fasting would help you do so. Indeed, in this study eating every other day was recommended as a treatment for asthma (lung inflammation).

What about stroke, heart disease, and heart attacks? In a 2017 review Dr. Longo wrote intermittent fasting

> **increased resistance of the brain and heart to stress via reduced tissue damage and improved function in models of stroke and heart disease.** Emerging findings are revealing cellular and molecular mechanisms by which IF increases the resistance of cells, tissues and organs to stress and common diseases associated with aging and sedentary lifestyles.[131]

---

[129] Johnson JB, et al. Alternate day calorie restriction improves clinical findings and reduces markers of oxidative stress and inflammation in overweight adults with moderate asthma. *Free Radic. Biol. Med.* 2007;42:665–674.
[130] Robbins T, Diamandis PH. *Life Force: How New Breakthroughs in Precision Medicine Can Transform the Quality of Your Life & Those You Love.* Simon and Schuster; 2022. pg 276
[131] Mattson MP, Longo VD, Harvie M. Impact of intermittent fasting on health and disease processes. *Ageing Research Reviews.* 2017;39:46-58. doi:10.1016/j.arr.2016.10.005

This means you could practice IF to lower risk of death by stroke or heart attack, regardless of diet and exercise, provided you do not overeat. Doing so would give you more years with the ones you love.

A 2020 study showed time-restricted feeding prevents weight gain, improves sleep, and mitigates age-related heart dysfunction while improving blood pressure and cholesterol.[132] Lowering the risk of heart attack with IF will grant you a longer, healthier life.

Anyone curious how much longer? Research shows an increase in BMI by two points shortens American life expectancy by one year.[133] This means you live longer with lower BMI via fasting. One animal study revealed that mice subjected to alternate-day fasting lived 30% longer.[134] They also exhibited delayed onset of age-related diseases.

Intermittent fasting can lower your risk of the top two causes of premature death: cardiovascular disease and cancer. By preventing the top causes of death, you can enjoy more years with people you love.

More longevity benefits for women

---

[132] Wilkinson MJ et al. Ten-hour time-restricted eating reduces weight, blood pressure, and atherogenic lipids in patients with metabolic syndrome. Cell Metab 31, 92–104 (2020).

[133] Peto R., Whitlock G., Jha P. Effects of obesity and smoking on U.S. life expectancy. *N. Engl. J. Med.* 2010;362(9):855–856. doi: 10.1056/NEJMc1000079.

[134] Anson RM, et al. Intermittent fasting dissociates beneficial effects of dietary restriction on glucose metabolism and neuronal resistance to injury from calorie intake. *Proceedings of the National Academy of Sciences of the United States of America*. 2003;100(10):6216-6220. doi:10.1073/pnas.1035720100

A 2016 review of women's health research showed fasting helps women over 50 in four ways: cancer prevention, metabolic health, mental health, and chronic pain from inflammation.[135] We already covered the anticancer benefits of IF. Regarding metabolic health, women over 50 show a higher prevalence for metabolic syndrome: increased abdominal fat, blood sugar and cholesterol. This review reinforced cardiovascular health benefits covered above:

> ... study results confirmed the **significant cardioprotective actions of IF**: weight loss; [lowered] fat, blood pressure, and heart rate; and decrease in total and LDL cholesterol.[136]

In other words, IF is anti-metabolic syndrome. In 2017 Dr. Longo co-authored a study involving 63 women on a fasting-mimicking diet (FMD) five days a month for three months. The results? It lowered weight, body fat, blood sugar, blood pressure, and cholesterol (total TG dropped 19 units).[137] Since FMD is done periodically, researchers also noted beneficial effects were maintained for months after subjects returned to their normal diet. **If you know a woman that wants to lose weight, improve metabolic syndrome, lower risk factors for death, or slow aging and reduce inflammation, she could incorporate short periods of FMD.**

---

[135] Nair PM, Khawale PG. Role of therapeutic fasting in women's health: An overview. J Midlife Health. 2016 Apr-Jun;7(2):61-4. doi: 10.4103/0976-7800.185325.
[136] Ibid
[137] Wei, M., et al. Fasting-mimicking diet and markers/risk factors for aging, diabetes, cancer, and cardiovascular disease. *Science Translational Medicine.* 2017;9(377). doi:10.1126/scitranslmed.aai8700

Research underscores the potential of a fasting-mimicking diet and time-restricted feeding for improved women's health and the time in which you are youthful, healthy and fully functional.[138]

Anti-aging benefits

Do you know women that want to look younger? In 2019 Dr. Longo authored a paper on periodic fasting and longevity. In it he explains fasting promotes a stress resistance state activating cell protection, regeneration, and rejuvenation.[139] He wrote

> ...these states can be viewed as a longevity program activated to [extend youth] via periodic cellular regeneration and autophagy in addition to chronic protection and repair.

This means periodic fasting slows aging and rejuvenates tissue.

A 2015 study found periodic fasting (FMD) can rejuvenate tissues and organs through the activation of cell death, autophagy, and stem cell activation.[140] Remember, your stem cells can become any needed cell in your body: heart, nerve, skin, immune cell etc. So **you want abundant stem cells for youthful looks and performance.** The refeeding period after fasting is your time for replacing damaged cells

[138] Longo VD. Programmed longevity, youthspan, and juventology. *Aging Cell*. 2018;18(1). doi:10.1111/acel.12843
[139] Ibid
[140] Brandhorst S et al. A periodic diet that mimics fasting promotes multi-system regeneration, enhanced cognitive performance, and healthspan. *Cell Metab*. 2015 Jul 7;22(1):86-99. doi: 10.1016/j.cmet.2015.05.012.

with tissue-specific stem cells.[141] This means **fasting activates stem cells to regenerate your tissue, boosting immunity!** A 2015 animal study showed three cycles of FMD increased lean muscle mass.[142] If you want to look leaner, you might use FMD. The same study showed three cycles of FMD reduces biomarkers of aging.

Do you want to improve wrinkles or immunity? Harvard research by Dr. Sinclair shows it's natural that your stem cells decline with age causing tissue damage and dysfunction. This can result in gray hair, wrinkles, and declining immunity. Repeated periods of FMD can partially revert age-related decline of stem cells to repair your tissues.[143] The skewing of your stem cells also contributes to declining immunity.[144] FMD has been scientifically shown to promote stem cell proliferation and regeneration of the immune system.[145] If you want to maintain robust immunity, research suggests multiple rounds of FMD.

Do you want to improve sleep, heart function, and reduce risk for metabolic syndrome? If so, eating all your calories in ten hours per day (TRF) may be the easiest method. A 2020 study on overweight patients showed 14:10 prevents excessive weight gain, improves sleep, slows deteriorating

[141] Cheng C-W et al. Prolonged fasting reduces IGF-1/PKA to promote hematopoietic-stem-cell-based regeneration and reverse immunosuppression. *Cell Stem Cell* 14, 810–823 (2014).

[142] Brandhorst S et al. A periodic diet that mimics fasting promotes multi-system regeneration, enhanced cognitive performance, and healthspan. *Cell Metab* 22, 86–99 (2015).

[143] Ibid

[144] Schultz MB & Sinclair DA. When stem cells grow old: phenotypes and mechanisms of stem cell aging. *Development* 143, 3–14 (2016).

[145] Cheng C-W et al. Prolonged fasting reduces IGF-1/PKA to promote hematopoietic-stem-cell-based regeneration and reverse immunosuppression. *Cell Stem Cell* 14, 810–823 (2014).

heart function, and lowers blood pressure and cholesterol.[146] Eating all calories in *six* hours a day comes with the added benefit of reduced oxidative stress.[147]

Speaking of beauty sleep and youthful appearance, chew on this. Research shows disrupting the circadian rhythm for ten days yields higher blood sugar, blood pressure, insulin resistance and fat.[148] If you want to live longer with more energy, you want to maintain a stable biological clock. In other words, try to avoid night shift work and changing your routine bedtime and wake up time (see Chapter 6).

Will IF work for you for slowing aging? Yes. An eight week time-restricted feeding study of 19 postmenopausal women showed good adherence to this lifestyle change with reduced body fat, insulin resistance, and oxidative stress.[149] In 2021 Dr. Longo wrote TRF periods of approximately 12 hours appear to be associated with benefits without side effects.[150] This suggests eating all food in 12 hours per day can help any woman with weight loss and slow aging.

---

[146] Wilkinson MJ et al. Ten-hour time-restricted eating reduces weight, blood pressure, and atherogenic lipids in patients with metabolic syndrome. *Cell Metab* 31, 92–104 (2020).

[147] Cienfuegos S, et al. Effects of 4- and 6-h time-restricted feeding on weight and cardiometabolic health: a randomized controlled trial in adults with obesity. *Cell Metab* 32, 366–378 (2020).

[148] Scheer FA, et al. Adverse metabolic and cardiovascular consequences of circadian misalignment. *Proc Natl Acad Sci U S A.* 2009;106:4453–4458.

[149] Cienfuegos S, et al. Changes in body weight and metabolic risk during time restricted feeding in premenopausal versus postmenopausal women. *Experimental Gerontology.* 2021;154:111545. doi:10.1016/j.exger.2021.111545

[150] Longo VD, et al. Intermittent and periodic fasting, longevity and disease. *Nature Aging.* 2021;1(1):47-59. doi:10.1038/s43587-020-00013-3

Leading research shows IF can increase your health and longevity at the cellular and clinical level. It activates autophagy for youthful performance, balances hormones, is anti-inflammatory, anti-oxidative stress, anti-heart disease and anti-cancer. This means IF can repair and rejuvenate your tissue while reducing risk of the top two causes of death. In other words, IF can slow aging for longer life. So fasting can increase the time you get to spend with people you love.

Reducing chronic pain in women over 50

Anyone you know suffering with chronic pain that only gets worse, causing disability? Prevalence of joint and bone health problems increase with age, according to a 2016 review of women's health.[151]

Fasting improves arthritis by reducing food intolerance, lowering gut permeability, and decreasing inflammatory proteins.[152] A study on arthritis patients fasting for 7–10 days and eating vegetarian showed decreased pain, stiffness, and dependence on painkillers.[153] This was observed in 1979! **If you want to reduce joint pain and painkiller costs, you could eat vegetarian and implement a seven day fast.**

---

[151] Nair, MKP, and Kawhale, PG. Role of therapeutic fasting in women's health: An overview. *J Midlife Health.* 2016 Apr-Jun; 7(2): 61–64. doi: 10.4103/0976-7800.185325
[152] Hafström I, et al. Effects of fasting on disease activity, neutrophil function, fatty acid composition, and leukotriene biosynthesis in patients with rheumatoid arthritis. *Arthritis Rheum.* 1988;31:585–92.
[153] Sköldstam L, Larsson L, Lindström FD. Effect of fasting and lactovegetarian diet on rheumatoid arthritis. *Scand J Rheumatol.* 1979;8:249–55.

In 2001 a review of four studies showed fasting periods lasting from 1 to 3 weeks reduce the symptoms of arthritis, although these effects are reversed by a return to the normal diet... unless the fast is followed by a vegetarian diet.[154]

Osteoporosis is the leading cause of bone fracture and falls in aging women. IF is shown to benefit bone health. Fasting affects the parathyroid hormone which plays a major role in both calcium and phosphate metabolism and the bone remodeling process.[155] IF-mediated weight loss also reduces risk of fracture from osteoporosis.

One study also showed a 24 hour fast before and after chemotherapy reduced bone marrow toxicity.[156] This means fasting helps bone health in even the most weakened state: in cancer patients receiving chemotherapy.

Intermittent fasting is shown to improve chronic pain in arthritis patients and lower risk of osteoporosis by improving bone health.

This chapter has a ton of credible information. Table 1 is a good summary of the key points in this chapter. Notice all intermittent fasting methods are proven to lose weight while reducing your risk factors for heart disease, the leading cause of death.

---

[154] H. Müller, F.W. de Toledo, K.-L. Resch. Fasting followed by vegetarian diet in patients with rheumatoid arthritis: a systematic review. Scand. J. Rheumatol., 30 (2001), pp. 1-10

[155] Fraser WD, et al. Alteration of the circadian rhythm of intact parathyroid hormone and serum phosphate in women with established postmenopausal osteoporosis. *Osteoporos Int.* 1998;8:121–6.

[156] Groot Sde, et al. The effects of short-term fasting on tolerance to (neo) adjuvant chemotherapy in HER2-negative breast cancer patients: a randomized pilot study. BMC Cancer. 2015;15:652 https://doi.org/10.1186%2Fs12885-015-1663-5

Table 1: Fasting and disease risk factors [157]

Fasting method	Decreased risk factors for heart disease death
Alternate-day fasting	Weight, total and LDL cholesterol, triglycerides, fat mass
5:2 is fasting just two days a week	Weight, insulin resistance
Time-restricted feeding, e.g. 16:8	Weight, fat, leptin, systolic blood pressure
FMD, usually five days of 500 calories per month	Weight, systolic blood pressure, total and LDL cholesterol, inflammation (CRP, IGF-1)

Studies on intermittent fasting provide compelling evidence for mental health, hormone balancing, gut health, anti-aging and longevity benefits for women over 50. At a cellular level intermittent fasting activates cellular stress response pathways, repairing oxidative stress and DNA damage, repair and rejuvenation of tissue (autophagy), hormonal changes, and lower inflammation. Fasting is also proven to prevent and reverse diabetes and lower risk factors for heart disease and cancer. This means intermittent fasting promotes healthy aging and increased lifespan. So if you want to perform younger, feel better, and live longer for more time with the people you love, you could use intermittent fasting.

---

[157] Amended from Longo VD, et al. Intermittent and periodic fasting, longevity and disease. *Nature Aging*. 2021;1(1):47-59. doi:10.1038/s43587-020-00013-3

In the next chapter you'll discover why fasting is effective for long term weight loss via metabolic switching. The following chapters will help you design a personalized fasting plan for you to reap the countless benefits of intermittent fasting.

Chapter 3

Metabolic Switching: The Secret Sauce to Sustainable Weight Loss

Burn Fat, Not Sugar!

We know calorie counting and increased exercise often result in temporary outcomes, with weight regain being a common issue. In 2001 an analysis of 29 scientific studies showed that within five years of losing weight about 80% of the weight comes back.[158]

In recent years, a new paradigm has emerged, highlighting the significance of metabolic switching as the missing link in sustainable weight loss. How about a proven method for losing over 20 lbs and keeping it off?

Understanding Metabolic Switching

Metabolic switching refers to the body's ability to transition between different energy sources for fuel. It involves shifting from burning sugar (carbohydrates) to burning fat (ketones). You will be burning sugar or fat for energy. This metabolic switch is regulated by various factors including when you eat (when you fast), hormonal balance, and exercise.

Dr. Mattson has been researching fasting for over 20 years, co-authoring several studies with Dr. Longo (our fasting and longevity expert from Chapter 2). He explains after hours

---

[158] Anderson JW, et al. Long-term weight-loss maintenance: a meta-analysis of US studies. Am J Clin Nutr 2001;74(5):579–584. doi: 10.1093/ajcn/74.5.579.

without food, the body exhausts its sugar stores and starts burning fat:

> Intermittent fasting contrasts with the normal eating pattern for most [Western diet consumers], who eat throughout their waking hours... If someone is eating three meals a day, plus snacks, and they're not exercising, then every time they eat, they're running on those [food] calories and not burning their fat stores.[159]

Intermittent fasting works because it gives the body more time to exhaust sugar reserves from the last meal and switch to burning fat. You must switch back and forth between sugar burning and fat burning as this is how your body is naturally designed.

The best way to switch to burning fat is not the keto diet. In fact, to maximize weight loss, you want to avoid refined carbohydrates eaten in a keto diet. Remember research shows carbs do not cause you to gain fat; eating refined carbs causes you to gain fat and is associated with obesity.[160] You also want to favor whole foods and avoid processed foods found in the keto diet, e.g. cheese.

---

[159] Intermittent Fasting: What is it, and how does it work? Johns Hopkins Medicine. Published September 29, 2023. https://www.hopkinsmedicine.org/health/wellness-and-prevention/intermittent-fasting-what-is-it-and-how-does-it-work#:~:text=Mattson%20says%20that%20after%20hours,waking%20hours%2C%E2%80%9D%20Mattson%20says

[160] Spadaro, P, et al. A refined high carbohydrate diet is associated with changes in the serotonin pathway and visceral obesity. *Genetics Research*. 2015;97. https://doi.org/10.1017/s0016672315000233

One more reason to avoid keto is in a review of 13 keto diet studies in the *British Journal of Nutrition*. This 2013 review found that the keto diet increases cholesterol (LDL cholesterol) over twelve months compared to a low fat diet.[161] For healthy, lasting weight loss women may choose to avoid keto. Women looking for the healthiest outcome might consider eating whole foods, plant-based. After all, there are two aspects of weight loss: how often you eat and what you eat. For more on the diet that can facilitate healthy weight and long life see *The Whole Foods Diet for Longevity*.

In 2018 Dr. Mattson co-authored a scientific journal article called "Flipping the Metabolic Switch: Understanding and Applying Health Benefits of Fasting." Leading research shows the metabolic switch represents an evolutionarily conserved trigger to switch from fat storage to fat burning. Dr. Mattson wrote "intermittent fasting regimens that induce the metabolic switch [can] improve body composition in overweight individuals."[162] This means intermittent fasting switches your metabolism to burn fat. This study shows your metabolic switch to fat burning is turned on after you stop eating for 12 straight hours.

Enhanced Metabolic Flexibility

Metabolic switching promotes metabolic flexibility; efficiently switching back and forth between sugar burning and fat burning. This flexibility allows the body to adapt to

---

[161] Bueno NB, et al. Very-low-carbohydrate ketogenic diet v. low-fat diet for long-term weight loss: a meta-analysis of randomised controlled trials. Br J Nutr. 2013;110(7):1178-1187. doi: 10.1017/S0007114513000548.

[162] Anton SD, et al. Flipping the metabolic switch: Understanding and applying the health benefits of fasting. *Obesity*. 2017;26(2):254-268. doi:10.1002/oby.22065

different nutritional states, such as fasting or variations in macronutrients, e.g. low fat, low protein, high carb.

If your goal is losing fat, you may think "I want to be in fat burning mode all the time." You could think that, but you'd be wrong. Don't forget that your whole brain and nervous system is primarily composed of fatty tissue (myelin nerve sheaths), and abdominal fat cushions organs and can keep you warm. Moreover, a lot of excess fat traps toxins that build up in your system to protect you. This means you do not want fat burning every day all day. Hence the reason we can metabolically switch from fat burning to sugar burning.

In a 2019 review of intermittent fasting research in the prestigious *New England Journal of Medicine*, Dr. Mattson wrote

> Periodic flipping of the metabolic switch not only provides the ketones [from burning fat] necessary to fuel [the body] during fasting, but also elicits highly orchestrated cellular responses that bolster mental and physical performance, as well as disease resistance.[163]

Dr. Mattson is saying that you must flip the metabolic switch on and off regularly via intermittent fasting to enjoy all the benefits, including burning fat.

---

[163] De Cabo R, Mattson MP. Effects of intermittent fasting on health, aging, and disease. *The New England Journal of Medicine.* 2019;381(26):2541-2551. doi:10.1056/nejmra1905136

Metabolic Switching for Burning Fat Long Term

"If you want to be successful [losing weight] you have to DECREASE hunger and INCREASE metabolic rate."[164]

-

- *Jason Fung, MD in lecture to other physicians about weight loss, bestselling author of The Obesity Code*

A 2016 study found that time-restricted feeding burned fat via increased fat oxidation and improved metabolic flexibility.[165] **In this study participants measured lower body fat in two months eating all calories in eight hours per day (16:8).** So you could lower your body fat by eating all daily food from 12pm - 8pm. Based on the research above, the 16 hour fasting window allows fat burning for four hours. IF works for weight loss in two months. What if you want to keep the weight off for longer than two months?

One 2022 study on women fasting two days a week lost 9% of their weight in three months.[166] This would be like a 200 lb woman losing nearly 20 lbs in three months without changing what she eats or exercise! Moreover, nearly 50% of the fasting women enjoyed over 10% weight loss versus only

---

[164] Jason Fung. Science of Intermittent Fasting | Intermittent Fasting | Jason Fung. *YouTube*. Published online July 17, 2022. https://www.youtube.com/watch?v=6aiR1mFD7Gw at 40:00

[165] Moro T, et al. Effects of eight weeks of time-restricted feeding (16/8) on basal metabolism, maximal strength, body composition, inflammation, and cardiovascular risk factors in resistance-trained males. *Journal of Translational Medicine*. 2016;14(1). doi:10.1186/s12967-016-1044-0

[166] Kang J, et al. Effects of an Intermittent Fasting 5:2 Plus Program on Body Weight in Chinese Adults with Overweight or Obesity: A Pilot Study. *Nutrients*. 2022;14(22):4734. doi:10.3390/nu14224734

14% in the calorie counting group. **This means 5:2 fasting was three times more effective for weight loss** than counting calories.

In a 2013 study of over 100 overweight women, one group did 5:2 IF and the other did calorie counting. The fasting groups showed lower waist size over six months and increased insulin sensitivity.[167] So **fasting just two days a week would drop inches off your waist and keep the weight off for six months.**

In 2019 a 12-month study of over 1400 people on a fasting-mimicking diet of 4-21 days enjoyed benefits just like a 5:2 regimen. It showed significant decreases in weight, waist size, blood pressure, blood sugar and increased ketones from the fasting-induced metabolic switch.[168] This suggests you could mimic fasting for just five days a month to switch to fat burning, losing inches off your waist.

Three cycles of FMD for five days every month for three months showed decreased biomarkers for aging, cardiovascular disease, and cancer. These included reduced weight, abdominal fat, blood pressure, cholesterol, and inflammation (IGF-1 and CRP).[169] So fasting five days a month would lose weight with the bonus of lower risk of heart disease death.

---

[167] Harvie M et al. The effect of intermittent energy and carbohydrate restriction v. daily energy restriction on weight loss and metabolic disease risk markers in overweight women. *Br. J. Nutr* 110, 1534–1547 (2013).
[168] Wilhelmi de Toledo F, et al. Safety, health improvement and well-being during a 4 to 21-day fasting period in an observational study including 1422 subjects. *PLoS ONE* 14, e0209353 (2019).
[169] Wei M, et al. Fasting-mimicking diet and markers/risk factors for aging, diabetes, cancer, and cardiovascular disease. *Science Translational Medicine.* 2017;9(377). doi:10.1126/scitranslmed.aai8700

Remember why fasting works from Dr. Fung: the metabolic rate goes up with IF without the hunger problems associated with calorie counting (see Introduction). This means IF would be sustainable for weight management because it does not lead to insulin resistance. **With low insulin levels you can flip the metabolic switch to fat burning.** Indeed, a 2021 study on 200 obese women practicing 5:2 IF showed they lost five pounds in six weeks and did not gain the weight back over twelve months.[170] This means **fasting two days a week keeps the weight off for 12 months via metabolic switching.** Everyone knows daily calorie counting leads to weight regain via high insulin and hunger.

In a simplified approach, a smartphone app to monitor what, when, and how much individuals eat has shed new light on eating patterns. Eight overweight people ate their normal daily calories within ten hours (14:10 IF). The eating window often ended past 8pm so that they could have dinner with family. They lost up to 4% body weight over four months and retained this weight loss for a year.[171] **In this study, a 200 lb woman would have lost 8 lbs in four months and kept it off for 12 months because of daily metabolic switching.** That's sustained weight loss with IF for a full year you do not get with yo-yo dieting, and it doesn't require changing what you eat or exercise.

It gets better. Did you know fasting is more effective for weight loss than changing the amount of fat in your diet? A 2020 study explored the metabolic response to a low

---

[170] Hájek P, et al. A randomised controlled trial of the 5:2 diet. *PLOS ONE*. 2021;16(11):e0258853. doi:10.1371/journal.pone.0258853
[171] Gill S, Panda S. A Smartphone App Reveals Erratic Diurnal Eating Patterns in Humans that Can Be Modulated for Health Benefits. *Cell Metabolism*. 2015;22(5):789-798. doi:10.1016/j.cmet.2015.09.005

carbohydrate, high fat (LCHF) diet in 57 middle aged obese women. Within ten weeks women eating LCHF lost 6.2 lbs.[172] **This study shows obese women can eat a high fat diet to lose weight.** Let me repeat that for emphasis: women can lose weight eating a high fat diet. However, *more* weight loss occurred two weeks faster eating normally for five days a week (5:2 IF). Why? The fasting flipped the metabolic switch from sugar burning five days a week to fat burning two days a week. This study proved fasting is superior to changing dietary carbs and fat for weight loss.

Here's a question for you: how do doctors lose weight? A 2020 study on 900 female doctors found they lost an average of 13.2 lbs in a year. The study showed 75% of them lost weight using IF.[173] This means IF was the most effective strategy for weight loss; more effective than keto diet (low carb) and calorie counting. **These highly educated women were asked to lose weight so they used the most effective method: intermittent fasting for metabolic switching to fat burning.** So IF is effective for losing weight and keeping it off for 12 months and you won't feel hungry like you do calorie counting. It's also empowering to know that you're using the proven most effective strategy.

Metabolic switching represents a crucial aspect of sustainable weight loss that is overlooked in traditional approaches like daily calorie counting and high-intensity

---

[172] Valsdottir TD, et al. Low-Carbohydrate High-Fat Diet and Exercise: Effect of a 10-Week Intervention on body Composition and CVD risk Factors in Overweight and Obese Women—A randomized controlled trial. *Nutrients*. 2020;13(1):110. doi:10.3390/nu13010110

[173] Hendrix JK, Aikens JE, Saslow LR. Dietary weight loss strategies for self and patients: A cross-sectional survey of female physicians. *Obesity Medicine*. 2020;17:100158. doi:10.1016/j.obmed.2019.100158

anaerobic exercise. By promoting fat burning through intermittent fasting, women can feel empowered and proud using metabolic switching for keeping weight off. You could also add aerobic exercise while fasting for more fat burning (see exercise below).

Abdominal Fat Secrets

Any women you know struggling with persistent belly fat? First and foremost, all fat is not the same. Remember belly fat accumulates over years of your body storing toxins and fat to protect and feed you. Research shows belly fat accumulates due to increased stress (cortisol levels).

A 1994 study on 41 overweight women showed cortisol levels increase 60 minutes after stress.[174] Stress naturally puts you in fight or flight mode. It's healthy to move soon after a stressful event because the immediate adrenaline release leads to increased cortisol within a couple hours.[175] **If you don't move under stress, there will be increased belly fat.** The authors wrote "cortisol secretion might represent a mechanism for the association between stress and abdominal fat."

Hold on. We've known for decades that increased stress increases belly fat? Yes. A 2000 study at Yale showed increased cortisol in overweight and healthy women increased abdominal fat (aka visceral fat).[176] Cortisol affects

---

[174] Moyer A, et al. Stress-Induced cortisol response and fat distribution in women. *Obesity Research*. 1994;2(3):255-262. doi:10.1002/j.1550-8528.1994.tb00055.x

[175] van der Valk ES, Savas M, van Rossum EFC. Stress and Obesity: Are There More Susceptible Individuals? Curr Obes Rep. 2018 Jun;7(2):193-203. doi: 10.1007/s13679-018-0306-y.

[176] Study: Stress may cause excess abdominal fat in otherwise slender. YaleNews. Published May 17, 2018.

fat distribution by causing fat to be stored around the organs. In other words, stress increases belly fat. People with diseases associated with extreme exposure to cortisol, like depression, have excessive amounts of abdominal fat.

Yale researchers wrote

> It is possible that greater exposure to stress in their daily lives [led to] greater lifetime exposure to cortisol. Cortisol may have caused them to accumulate abdominal fat.[177]

That's Yale saying increased stress can cause increased belly fat. Menopause is very stressful physically and emotionally. So is raising teenagers and babysitting grandkids. Other stressors that may come up after menopause include sleep deprivation (see Chapter 6) and chronic pain and inflammation (see Chapter 2).

A 2017 analysis showed chronic stress is associated with a 22% increase in cortisol.[178] In addition, a 2016 study showed obese people experiencing discrimination had higher cortisol levels than obese people who did not feel discrimination.[179] **Weight discrimination can increase obesity by increasing cortisol**, **which is associated with increased belly fat.** It's a vicious cycle where obese

---

https://news.yale.edu/2000/09/22/study-stress-may-cause-excess-abdominal-fat-otherwise-slender-women
[177] Ibid
[178] Stalder T, et al. Stress-related and basic determinants of hair cortisol in humans: a meta-analysis. *Psychoneuroendocrinology*. 2017;77:261–274.
[179] Jackson SE, Kirschbaum C, Steptoe A. Perceived weight discrimination and chronic biochemical stress: A population-based study using cortisol in scalp hair. *Obesity*. 2016;24(12):2515-2521. doi:10.1002/oby.21657

women experience stress which intensifies obesity. So you want to lower stress to lower weight.

Maximum belly fat loss in one month

In 2019 the largest clinical trial to date showed a variant of alternate day fasting burned primarily abdominal fat.[180] The fasting cycles were defined as strict 36 hour fasts followed by 12 hour eating windows for 30 days. In the 12 hour eating days they ate whatever they wanted and still enjoyed massive weight loss. This 36 hour fast alternated with one normal eating day keeps you in belly fat burning mode for 30 days! This would give you **the fastest, greatest abdominal fat loss in a month based on science and it's free.** These people lost 4.5% of their weight, mostly belly fat, in a month. For a 200 lb woman that's losing 10 lbs in a month naturally, for free.

Please note the best fasting method for you is the one you can sustain month in and month out. It's not recommended for beginners to go straight for this 36 hour fasting protocol. This is for overweight people struggling to lose weight long term with fasting experience, who are slowly increasing their fasting hours over time. For weight loss protocols and strategies proven for women see Chapter 6.

Metabolic Switching and IF in Women over 50

Understanding metabolic switching in women is crucial, as their hormonal profiles and metabolic responses differ from men. Men have only testosterone. Women have three sex hormones: estrogen, progesterone, and testosterone. With

---

[180] Stekovic S, et al. Alternate day fasting improves physiological and molecular markers of aging in healthy, non-obese humans. *Cell Metabolism.* 2019;30(3):462-476.e6. doi:10.1016/j.cmet.2019.07.016

menopause, your estrogen and progesterone levels drop and you no longer ovulate. The decrease in estrogen may lead to symptoms like vaginal dryness, mood changes, night sweats and hot flashes.

Hormonal Influence on Metabolic Switching

Research suggests time-restricted feeding would help postmenopausal women with insulin levels to keep weight off, reducing body fat, insulin resistance, and chronic inflammation. **A 2021 study on 15 women with no menstrual cycle showed hormone improvements in five weeks of eating eight hours a day:** testosterone, insulin, and a protein that binds estrogen.[181] Remember, when insulin stays low by fasting long enough, you switch to fat burning. Bonus effects included lower weight, body fat, abdominal fat, and inflammation. The same IF intervention improved cycle regularity in 73% of women. Yes, you heard that right! For 11/15 women, IF restored their menstrual cycle by improving hormone levels.

Feel free to review Chapter 2 for more on hormone balancing and weight loss. Foods to support your hormones and weight loss are detailed in Chapter 4.

How to Exercise for Fat Burning

Remember the 2023 review that stated the most effective fat loss strategy is combining fasting and exercise?[182] This

---

[181] Li C, et al. Eight-hour time-restricted feeding improves endocrine and metabolic profiles in women with anovulatory polycystic ovary syndrome. *Journal of Translational Medicine*. 2021;19(1). doi:10.1186/s12967-021-02817-2

[182] Eglseer D, et al. Nutrition and Exercise Interventions to Improve Body Composition for Persons with Overweight or Obesity Near Retirement Age: A Systematic Review and Network Meta-Analysis of Randomized

means you could get better results adding exercise to your fasting. Here you will discover how to exercise for fat burning and when to exercise for maximum results. Before showing you how, let me ask a few questions to see if they resonate with you. Have you ever put off exercise then when you finally do you push too hard, making up for lost time? Have you ever pushed yourself really hard in the gym for little to no benefit over a few months or years? One big knowledge gap regarding exercise and fat loss is that burning fat is done by conditioning the body to burn fat. In other words, **you must do aerobic exercise to burn fat.**

According to Dr. Maffetone, all exercise programs require you to begin by building an aerobic base during which you do no anaerobic exercise for two to eight months.[183] Aerobic exercise is moderate activity at a training heart rate of 180 - your age, per Stu Mittleman, and Dr. Maffetone.[184] This heart rate is recommended for fat burning by Stu Mittleman, famous for setting the world record running 1000 miles in eleven days. Stu Mittleman did something many say is impossible by mastering aerobic exercise.

If you want to burn fat during exercise, Mittleman recommends a 15 minute warmup at a low heart rate to mobilize the fatty acids to the blood.[185] **If you skip the**

Controlled Trials. *Advances in Nutrition*. 2023;14(3):516-538. doi:10.1016/j.advnut.2023.04.001

[183] See Chapter 13 in Maffetone P. *The Big Book of Health and Fitness: A Practical Guide to Diet, Exercise, Healthy Aging, Illness Prevention, and Sexual Well-Being*. Skyhorse Publishing Inc.; 2012. cited in Robbins T. *Awaken the Giant Within* pg 441 - 443

[184] Robbins T. *Awaken the Giant Within: How to Take Immediate Control of Your Mental, Emotional, Physical & Financial Destiny!*; 1991. pg 439 - 448

[185] Ibid

warmup you may use oxygen via aerobic exercise but not burn fat.

For example, the warmup HR at 50 would be 85 bpm. The warmup intensity is so low that it will feel like you're doing nothing, barely more intense than standing still. According to Mittleman you then train at a HR of 130 bpm (180 - your age). He recommends starting with aerobic training for at least 20 minutes three times a week. Dr. Maffetone suggests doing this exclusively for two to eight months, before adding anaerobic exercise.

You would rate the intensity of aerobic exercise around 6/10 - 7/10 with minimal sweat. Here's a simple test to see if you're aerobic: if you can carry out a conversation while exercising without being short of breath it's aerobic. If you are short of breath talking during exercise it's anaerobic. Moderate level activities like walking are aerobic. Walking outside also reduces amygdala stimulation and moves your lymph fluid to carry waste and toxins away from tissue.[186] Do you want to detox? Go for a walk outside. This causes you to feel relaxed and a sense of well-being, and if it's a moderate walk it can burn fat. Better yet, you can walk to burn fat on just one piece of equipment: a treadmill or elliptical. Everything else you see at the gym is not required to burn fat.

A lot of people exercise at heart rates that are too high and burn sugar instead of fat by doing anaerobic exercise. Some examples of anaerobic exercise include sprinting, speed cycling, and high intensity interval

_____

[186] Sudimac S, Sale V, Kühn S. How nature nurtures: Amygdala activity decreases as the result of a one-hour walk in nature. *Molecular Psychiatry*. 2022;27(11):4446-4452. doi:10.1038/s41380-022-01720-6

training (HIIT). If you maintain a heart rate of over 180 - your age, you are doing anaerobic exercise.[187] For example, if you are 50 exercising over 130 bpm your heart rate is too high. This trains your body to burn sugar instead of fat. **This is why so many women are obsessed with losing the last 10 lbs of fat.** If you train your body to burn sugar, changing your eating habits (IF and/or diet change) may not yield maximum weight loss. You can exercise aerobically as described below to burn fat instead of sugar. Make sure to use an accurate heart rate monitor, e.g. WHOOP strap, FitBit, Apple watch, etc.

Table 1 shows you calculated heart rates for your warmup and aerobic training (i.e. heart rate to burn fat). You will see the warmup heart rate is [(220 - age) / 2] as usual. **The fat burning heart rate is based on Mittleman's results running over 80 miles a day for eleven days, a feat most personal trainers would say is impossible.** The aerobic training heart rate is 180 - your age. Remember to train at this heart rate for at least 20 minutes.

Table 1: Warmup and aerobic training heart rates (HR to burn fat) for each decade.

Age (y)	Warmup HR (15 min)	HR to burn fat (20 min+)
50	85 bpm	130 bpm
60	80 bpm	120 bpm
70	75 bpm	110 bpm
80	70 bpm	100 bpm

---

[187] Robbins T. *Awaken the Giant Within: How to Take Immediate Control of Your Mental, Emotional, Physical & Financial Destiny!*; 1991. pg 439-448

You can see the aerobic heart rates decrease with age and they are based on Stu Mittleman's formula for real, stunning results. Per Dr. Maffetone, if you have been ill or injured the past two years, reduce the heart rates by 5 bpm.[188] Remember if you skip the 15 minute warmup you will do aerobic exercise and not burn fat. **This plan would be even more effective after fasting for 12 hours based on Dr. Mattson's fasting research.** It's called training in the fasted state.

If you want maximum fat loss in minimum time, you could schedule your aerobic exercise *before* you eat a meal. This is called fast, train, eat. For example, if you are 50 you could fast for 12 hours by not eating after dinner, then do your 15 minute warm up at 85 bpm in the morning. Then train aerobically by walking for 20 minutes at 130 bpm. Then eat your meal. Doing this would start your aerobic exercise, primed to burn fat with sufficient warmup, after your body has already flipped the metabolic switch to burn fat.

Since metabolic switching to burning fat is controlled by hormones, **you might ask does training in the fasted state work with hormones?** Yes. Near the end of your fast, your adrenalin and growth hormone levels are high because insulin levels are low. This optimizes muscle function during training in a way that you can train harder. You heard that right: **you can train harder while fasting. Growth hormone levels are high so you can also enjoy faster recovery.**

When I train in the fasted state, I will do aerobic exercise in the morning before eating my first meal. I can tell you from

---

[188] Ibid

experience that I can train longer and harder. This is because when fasting I have *more* energy than training after eating.

NB: If you take medication you should consult your doctor before making exercise changes. Before changing my exercise plan I always consult my Doctor of Osteopathic Medicine (DO). I choose a DO instead of an MD because DOs have more training in lifestyle medicine.

Metabolic switching is a powerful tool for sustainable weight loss in women over 50. Research shows women can achieve weight loss, belly fat loss, lower body fat percentage, and improved metabolic health through intermittent fasting. If you want faster results, you can add aerobic training in the fasted state. By understanding and implementing metabolic switching, you can achieve sustainable weight loss and improved health. When you're ready to implement fasting for lasting weight loss, move on to Part II in this book, and see the customizable fasting plans and insights in Chapter 6.

Make a Difference with Your Review

Unlock the Secret to Weight Loss after Menopause

"The simplest rule of weight loss is just don't eat all the time... don't eat between this hour and this hour." - Dr. Jason Fung

I hope this message finds you well and ready to make a real impact. This book was written to make lasting weight loss a reality for every woman, and you play a crucial role in that journey.

People who give without expectation live longer, happier lives. Here's a question for you:

Would you help someone you've never met, even if you never got credit for it?

That someone is a woman like you, or perhaps like you used to be, wanting to make a difference and seeking guidance. Your generosity can be a beacon of light for her.

Why? Because your review can change lives.

My goal is to help every woman optimize weight, health, and longevity, and your review helps us get there. Most people judge a book by its cover and reviews.

This is where you come in. Picture a woman struggling with healthy weight after menopause. Your review could be the turning point in her life.

Your gift costs no money and takes less than 60 seconds to make real, but it can change a fellow woman's life forever.

Your review could:

- Help a woman you know lose weight and keep it off.
- Help another woman with mental clarity and memory.
- Help another woman with her health and longevity.
- Make one more dream come true.

To make a real difference and get that 'feel good' feeling, all you have to do is leave a review.

Simply scan the QR code below to leave your review:

If you're someone who feels good about helping a faceless woman struggling with weight and optimal health, welcome to the club. You're one of us.

I'm excited to share proven strategies for lasting weight loss in the chapters ahead.

Thank you from the bottom of my heart. Now, back to our regularly scheduled programming.

- Your biggest fan, Paul Griggs

PS - Fun fact: If you provide something of value to another person, it makes you more valuable to them. If you'd like goodwill straight from another woman—and you believe this book will help her—send this book her way.

Part II: The Art of Fasting Like a Woman

Chapter 4

Designing a Fasting Lifestyle Built and Sustainable for You

Fasting is flexible. If it's holidays you might say I'm not fasting, but then after the holidays I'm gonna do a lot of fasting because you gained weight. You can change the fasting duration or frequency and it applies to any diet. It's always up to you. It really offers unlimited power. [189]

- *Jason Fung, MD in lecture to other physicians on fasting and weight loss, bestselling author of The Obesity Code*

Dr. Mattson's extensive fasting research shows that it can take two to four weeks before the body becomes accustomed to intermittent fasting. You might feel hungry or cranky while you're getting used to the new routine. That said, research shows subjects who make it through the adjustment period tend to stick with it because they feel better.[190]

It's important to tailor a fasting lifestyle to your goals and preferences. This chapter focuses on designing a fasting

---

[189] Jason Fung. Science of Intermittent Fasting | Intermittent Fasting | Jason Fung. *YouTube*. Published online July 17, 2022. https://www.youtube.com/watch?v=6aiR1mFD7Gw at 44:38

[190] Intermittent Fasting: What is it, and how does it work? Johns Hopkins Medicine. Published September 29, 2023. https://www.hopkinsmedicine.org/health/wellness-and-prevention/intermittent-fasting-what-is-it-and-how-does-it-work#:~:text=Mattson%20says%20that%20after%20hours,waking%20hours%2C%E2%80%9D%20Mattson%20says

lifestyle unique to you, taking into account your routine and goals. By customizing your fasting approach, you can achieve your desired results long term. For example, if you are fasting to lose fat, to keep the weight off you will want to build a weekly fasting routine. This way you keep signaling your body to burn fat long term. You may also consider increasing hormone balancing foods (see below).

Assess Your Schedule and Lifestyle

To determine when not to eat, consider your daily routine, work schedule, and social commitments. Assess which fasting patterns align best with your lifestyle and allow for consistency. Consistent structured eating builds habits. Why do you want your fasting regimen to be a habit? **A weight loss habit requires no willpower.**

Remember in the 1970s we had a structured meal plan eating three meals a day, and many people rushing to work skipped breakfast, eating only lunch and dinner. They never ate between meals - no snacks! This means they benefited from intermittent fasting as a habit. They didn't have to think about incorporating fasting because it was normal to stop eating after dinner. In turn, **obesity was almost non-existent in the 1970s whereas it runs rampant now with people eating three meals plus snacks every day.**[191] This habit of overeating breakfast, lunch, dinner, snack is causing weight gain.

The most popular IF regimen is time-restricted feeding, starting with 12-14 hour fasts after dinner and building from

---

[191] Temple NJ. The origins of the obesity epidemic in the USA–Lessons for today. *Nutrients*. 2022;14(20):4253. doi:10.3390/nu14204253

there. The easiest way to extend the fast would be to skip breakfast. If you skip breakfast you may also benefit from sleeping 30 minutes longer.

Should you start fasting by skipping breakfast or dinner?

If you're new to fasting you don't want to go from eating three meals over 12 hours to eating in a six hour window, or every other day. That would be asking too much of yourself.

Women just starting out would find skipping breakfast is easier. Skipping dinner would be more effective for weight loss because it's usually the biggest meal. Fasting from lunch would signal the body via lower insulin to start burning fat long before going to sleep. While this will extend the time you are burning fat, it will be much harder to fit into your lifestyle because dinner is often a big, social gathering. You may have dinner with your family or friends. Skipping breakfast is easier because it's less social and you feel the least hungry in the morning.

Science shows people are hungriest at 8pm and least hungry at 8am.[192] You will feel the least hunger after waking up because hormones start waking the body before you rise. Growth hormone and cortisol levels peak only minutes before waking up (a regular fasting period) while hunger hormone levels are lower.[193] Breakfast, often associated with morning time when you're least hungry, is the smallest meal,

[192] Scheer FA, Morris CJ, Shea SA. The internal circadian clock increases hunger and appetite in the evening independent of food intake and other behaviors. Obesity (Silver Spring). 2013 Mar;21(3):421-3. doi: 10.1002/oby.20351.
[193] Kim TW, Jeong JH, Hong SC. The impact of sleep and circadian disturbance on hormones and metabolism. Int J Endocrinol. 2015;2015:591729. doi: 10.1155/2015/591729.

typically not social, and easy to skip for busy women who have to hit the day running. If you don't feel hungry in the morning, you do not have to eat. Remember breakfast means "break your fast." When you break your fast is your choice. You could break your fast in the morning, at 1pm at lunch, or you could break your fast at dinner, or the next day. When you break your fast is up to you.

If you want to lose weight and look your best ASAP, you might choose to skip dinner. Whether you skip dinner or eat dinner, you will not feel hungry after waking up because your hormones are priming your body to start your day with energy before you're awake. Perhaps you are getting ready for a wedding or a trip to the beach. Maybe you decide to compensate for inevitable overeating on your trip by increasing extended fasting periods before and after (see below).

Please note one study on Americans in the early nineties showed an association between skipping breakfast and increased mortality.[194] However, these people self-reported how often they skipped breakfast. Here is Dr. Longo's perspective: "epidemiological data are not easy to interpret and the association between daily fasting periods and increased incidence of disease could be explained by factors other than the fasting."[195] Dr. Longo is our fasting and longevity expert from Chapter 2. He is saying take that study

---

[194] Rong S, Snetselaar L, Xu G, et al. Association of skipping breakfast with cardiovascular and All-Cause mortality. *Journal of the American College of Cardiology*. 2019;73(16):2025-2032. doi:10.1016/j.jacc.2019.01.065

[195] Longo VD, et al. Intermittent and periodic fasting, longevity and disease. *Nature Aging*. 2021;1(1):47-59. doi:10.1038/s43587-020-00013-3

with a grain of salt.

Your fasting routine

To add fasting to your lifestyle, it's important to build a routine daily, weekly, and annually. Your daily routine would be easy to follow if you make a simple rule: "I decide not to eat after dinner." This will give your body the benefits of 12 hours of fasting every day. You might also have a rule that says "I decide not to eat before noon." In other words, skip breakfast. That would get you to 16:8, a popular TRF regimen for fat burning daily. Once that becomes a habit, you can speed up your results by varying the fasting periods weekly (see Chapter 6).

How about your annual routine? Remember there are also seasons of eating habits. Many people indulge over the holidays from Thanksgiving to Christmas and gain weight. You might plan for this inevitability and compensate with your yearly routine. Perhaps you decide to not fast over the holidays then the first week of January eat clean (i.e. no more refined carbs in desserts like pie and Christmas cookies). In January you could have a rule to resume your fasting schedule that you discontinued the previous five weeks. Remember fasting is flexible: **you are always in full control. Fasting should make you feel empowered.** Being flexible with your fasting can prevent feelings of food deprivation, increasing adherence over the long term.

Everyone responds differently to fasting. Experiment with different fasting patterns and durations to find what works best for you. Some people may thrive with shorter daily fasting windows, while others may prefer longer periods. Continually assess how you feel, your energy levels, and weight changes to fine-tune your fasting lifestyle.

Listen to Your Body

Feeling lightheaded or dizzy

If you feel lightheaded or a bit dizzy when you fast you're probably dehydrated. Make sure you're drinking enough water: 2.5-3.5L per day as recommended in *The European Journal of Nutrition*.[196] You can add natural flavors to the water, e.g. lemon, lime, and cucumber. The rind will release oils into the water that give it flavor and may reduce the hunger wave intensity when starting your fast.

Excessive urination and diarrhea

This may happens because as you fast insulin drops and the body holds on to less water (insulin tends to make the body hold on to water). If you are water fasting and have excessive urination or diarrhea you might want to try dry fasting for under 24 hours. The good news is if you do a dry fast you may feel less hungry than fasting with water.[197]

Headaches and constipation

You could add some sea salt to water to prevent mild headaches. If that's insufficient you could add zero calorie beverages with more flavor like black coffee, green tea, and herbal tea. Herbal tea is recommended after lunch if you are

---

[196] Perrier ET, et al. Hydration for health hypothesis: a narrative review of supporting evidence. *European Journal of Nutrition*. 2020;60(3):1167-1180. doi:10.1007/s00394-020-02296-z
[197] Jason Fung. 8 Fasting Variations for Weight Loss | Jason Fung. *YouTube*. Published online September 12, 2021. https://www.youtube.com/watch?v=GNUSFaQIIjg at 3:40

having trouble with water only fasting, especially since it is decaf. For more on caffeine and optimal sleep for weight loss see Chapter 6. Dr. Fung recommends using psyllium husk or taking a laxative if you experience constipation.

Feeling hungry

If you find flavored water and tea are not helping with hunger when you start fasting, you could try fat fasting. A lot of people find adding MCT oil to coffee is satiating. Many people are used to daily coffee. If you add MCT oil it helps you not break your fast so it may help you lose weight.[198] You might also try a fiber fast. This could be chia seeds only during fasting periods, e.g. 1 Tbsp seeds in a cup of water. High fiber foods keep you feeling full in small quantities (see fiber foods below).

Designing a fasting lifestyle unique to you involves considering your schedule, goals, and responses to fasting. Fasting is flexible and your approach will be tailor made by you for you. You heard that right: **you will feel determined and flexible as you build your own fasting schedule.** By making your own rules about when to eat and when to fast, you can create a sustainable, personalized fasting routine daily and weekly. Remember to consult with healthcare professionals if you take medication.

Foods to Support Hormones

Since fasting for weight loss signals your hormones to burn fat and regulate appetite, you may want to eat hormone balancing foods. You can find them in any grocery store.

---

[198] Ibid at 7:00

Notice hormone balancing foods are plant-based, in line with recommendations in Book 1 in this series.

Whole Grains

Foods like brown rice, quinoa and oatmeal provide fiber and nutrients that can be beneficial for hormonal health. According to a 2009 nutrition journal study, whole grains are associated with lower belly fat.[199]

Cruciferous Vegetables

Several studies show cruciferous vegetables like broccoli, cabbage, and kale, contain compounds known as I3C and diindolylmethane.[200] These compounds have been shown to modulate estrogen metabolism by reducing harmful estrogens (estrogen dominance).

Broccoli, cabbage, and Brussels sprouts contain I3C and sulforaphane, which have been shown to support estrogen metabolism.[201] Research indicates an increase in the ratio of a protective estrogen metabolite to a potentially harmful estrogen metabolite, positively affecting estrogen metabolism.[202]

---

[199] McKeown NM, et al. Whole-Grain Intake and Cereal Fiber Are Associated with Lower Abdominal Adiposity in Older Adults. *Journal of Nutrition*. 2009;139(10):1950-1955. doi:10.3945/jn.108.103762
[200] Reed GA, et al. A Phase I study of Indole-3-Carbinol in women: tolerability and effects. *Cancer Epidemiology, Biomarkers & Prevention*. 2005;14(8):1953-1960. doi:10.1158/1055-9965.epi-05-0121
[201] Higdon, J. V., et al. Cruciferous vegetables and human cancer risk: epidemiologic evidence and mechanistic basis. *Pharmacological Research*. 2007;55(3):224-236. doi:10.1016/j.phrs.2007.01.009.
[202] Michnovicz JJ, Adlercreutz H, Bradlow HL. Changes in levels of urinary estrogen metabolites after oral indole-3-carbinol treatment in

Nuts and Seeds

These are rich in omega 3 fats, vitamins, and minerals that support overall health, including hormone balance.[203] A 2018 study investigated the effects of flaxseed consumption on hormone levels in postmenopausal women. The findings demonstrated an increase in a sex hormone-binding protein (SHBG), which can help regulate estrogen levels and support hormonal balance.[204] Flaxseed can also lower primary estrogen (E1) levels for lower breast cancer risk in postmenopausal women.[205]

Flaxseeds are rich in lignans, a phytoestrogen that exhibits estrogenic, antioxidant and anti-inflammatory properties.[206] Flaxseed is shown to reduce atherosclerotic plaques from high cholesterol by 46%.[207] So seeds are shown to balance estrogen and improve cholesterol plaque buildup in blood vessels. On top of balancing estrogen, seeds could improve cholesterol and blood pressure as a bonus.

humans. J Natl Cancer Inst. 1997;89(10):718-723. doi: 10.1093/jnci/89.10.718.

[203] Kris-Etherton PM, et al. The role of tree nuts and peanuts in the prevention of coronary heart disease: multiple potential mechanisms. *Journal of Nutrition.* 2008;138(9):1746S-1751S. doi:10.1093/jn/138.9.1746s

[204] Jenabian N, Moghadam MJ, Homayouni F. The effect of flaxseed on sex hormone-binding globulin levels in postmenopausal women. J Menopausal Med. 2018;24(1):29-34. doi: 10.6118/jmm.2018.24.1.29.

[205] Sturgeon S.R., et al. Effect of dietary flaxseed on serum levels of estrogens and androgens in postmenopausal women. *Nutr. Cancer.* 2008;60:612–618. doi: 10.1080/01635580801971864.

[206] Prasad K, Mantha SV, Muir AD, Westcott ND. Reduction of hypercholesterolemic atherosclerosis by CDC-flaxseed with very low alpha-linolenic acid. *Atherosclerosis.* 1998;136(2):367-375. doi:10.1016/s0021-9150(97)00239-6

[207] Ibid

Soy

Soy foods like soymilk, sprouts, edamame and tofu are rich in phytoestrogens, with mild estrogen-like effects.[208]

Optimizing Estrogen through Diet

A 2023 study stated falling estrogen levels around menopause lead to a significant increase in total fat and abdominal obesity.[209] The study stated "estrogen has shown beneficial effects on weight control, fat distribution, and insulin resistance." How? Your estrogen regulates appetite and how much you burn sugar (glucose) as well as energy levels (mitochondrial function). It also facilitates maintenance of bone density and cardiovascular health.

As estrogen levels naturally decline after menopause, women may have symptoms like hot flashes, vaginal dryness, and bone loss. Bone density is the limiting factor to building lean muscle and as it declines can yield osteoporosis, fractures and falls.[210] **Research shows five nutrients benefit estrogen**: cruciferous vegetables, fiber, omega 3s,

[208] Anderson, J. W., et al. Meta-Analysis of the effects of soy protein intake on serum lipids. *The New England Journal of Medicine.* 1995;333(5):276-282. doi:10.1056/nejm199508033330502

[209] Zhu J, et al. Role of estrogen in the regulation of central and peripheral energy homeostasis: from a menopausal perspective. Ther Adv Endocrinol Metab. 2023 Sep 15;14:20420188231199359. doi: 10.1177/20420188231199359.

[210] For more on bone density and osteogenic loading see Robbins T, Diamandis PH. *Life Force: How New Breakthroughs in Precision Medicine Can Transform the Quality of Your Life & Those You Love.* Simon and Schuster; 2022. pg 330-333

antioxidants, and phytochemicals.[211] We just reviewed cruciferous vegetables.

Fiber

Dietary fiber has been associated with improved estrogen metabolism. High fiber foods include whole foods like berries, nuts and whole grains.[212] One study found that higher fiber intake was correlated with increased levels of SHBG, a protein that binds to estrogen, reducing its availability.[213] By increasing SHBG levels, dietary fiber can help regulate estrogen activity and balance in overweight women.

Omega 3s

A 2020 study in the journal *Nutrients* found three types of foods help estrogen balance including omega 3 fats, antioxidants, and phytochemicals.[214] A 2003 study demonstrated that omega-3 fatty acids can alter estrogen metabolism for a healthier estrogen balance.[215]

Which omega-3s do you want for estrogen balance? While you can get EPA and DHA from seafood, what you want most

---

[211] Ko SH, Kim H. Menopause-Associated Lipid Metabolic Disorders and Foods Beneficial for postmenopausal women. *Nutrients*. 2020;12(1):202. doi:10.3390/nu12010202
[212] For fiber foods see Chapter 3 in *The Whole Foods Diet for Longevity*
[213] Lu LJ, et al. Effects of soya consumption for one month on steroid hormones in premenopausal women: implications for breast cancer risk reduction. Cancer Epidemiol Biomarkers Prev. 1996 Jun;5(6):63-70.
[214] Ko SH, Kim H. Menopause-Associated Lipid Metabolic Disorders and Foods Beneficial for postmenopausal women. *Nutrients*. 2020;12(1):202. doi:10.3390/nu12010202
[215] Bagga D, et al. Effects of a very low fat, high fiber diet on serum hormones and menstrual function implications for breast cancer prevention. *Cancer*. 1995;76(12):2491-2496. doi:10.1002/1097-0142(19951215)76:12

is essential omega 3s (ALA); healthy fats not made by your body. All ALA foods are plant foods. The best sources of omega-3 ALA are walnuts, chia seeds, flaxseed, soy and canola oil.[216] Flaxseed balances estrogen in three ways.

Antioxidants

Foods richest in antioxidants are all plant-based foods and they will help balance estrogen. According to a 2020 study in the journal *Nutrients,* antioxidants reduce damage to protein and DNA and reduce inflammation in obesity, metabolic syndrome, diabetes, high blood pressure, and high cholesterol.[217] This means postmenopausal diseases like metabolic syndrome are preventable with antioxidant foods that balance estrogen.

Foods richest in antioxidants for estrogen balance are spices, berries, and nuts, and all plant foods are high in antioxidants (see Table 1). Foods high in vitamin A, C, and E are also high in antioxidants.[218] You may decide to avoid foods lowest in antioxidants like meat, dairy and seafood (see Table 1).

Table 1: Food ranked by antioxidant content, from Nutrition Journal 2010.[219]

———————————————

[216] For omega 3 ALA foods see Chapter 3, Table 3 in *The Whole Foods Diet for Longevity* and section 4.2.5 in Ko SH, Kim H. Menopause-Associated Lipid Metabolic Disorders and Foods Beneficial for postmenopausal women. *Nutrients.* 2020;12(1):202. doi:10.3390/nu12010202

[217] Ko SH, Kim H. Menopause-Associated Lipid Metabolic Disorders and Foods Beneficial for postmenopausal women. *Nutrients.* 2020;12(1):202. doi:10.3390/nu12010202

[218] For more on antioxidant vitamin foods see Chapter 3 in *The Whole Foods Diet for Longevity*

[219] See Table 1 in Carlsen, M et al. The total antioxidant content of more than 3100 foods, beverages, spices, herbs and supplements used worldwide. Nutr J. 2010 Jan 22;9:3. doi: 10.1186/1475-2891-9-3.

Rank	Food	Antioxidant content (mmol/100g serving)
1	Spices and herbs	29.02
2	Berries and berry products	9.86
3	Nuts and seeds	4.57
4	Fruit and fruit juices	1.25
5	Breakfast cereals	1.09
6	Vegetables	0.80
7	Fats and oils	0.51
8	Legumes	0.48
9	Grains and grain products	0.34
10	Meat and meat products	0.31
11	Poultry	0.23
12	Dairy products	0.14

| 13 | Fish and seafood | 0.11 |
| 14 | Egg | 0.04 |

Phytochemicals

Phytochemicals are plant nutrients containing bioactive compounds to improve physiology. These include flavonoids, carotenoids, and tannins. Several function as antioxidants, which protect DNA, lipids, and other cellular components from oxidative stress.[220] Some can regulate protein synthesis, mimic hormones, and affect blood chemistry.

For flavonoids, you can have vegetables, fruits, nuts, whole grains, spices, and dark chocolate. Colorful carotenoids are in fruit and vegetables: cantaloupe, tomatoes, broccoli, carrots, pumpkin, spinach, and sweet potatoes. Notice broccoli helps estrogen in two ways: as a cruciferous vegetable also rich in phytochemicals.

Polyphenols function as phytoestrogens and are highly concentrated in grape skin and wine, known as resveratrol.[221] So grapes are another fruit to balance estrogen.

---

[220] Ko SH, Kim H. Menopause-Associated Lipid Metabolic Disorders and Foods Beneficial for postmenopausal women. *Nutrients*. 2020;12(1):202. doi:10.3390/nu12010202
[221] Gehm BD, et al. Resveratrol, a polyphenolic compound found in grapes and wine, is an agonist for the estrogen receptor. *Proceedings of*

Optimizing Progesterone through Diet

Progesterone, an essential hormone for women's health, plays a vital role in overall hormonal balance, often associated with feeling calm, rather than irritable or anxious. After menopause, progesterone levels drop. High carb foods and omega 3s help balance progesterone.

Progesterone foods

These include nuts and seeds, beans, and high carbohydrate foods like whole grains, potatoes, and cruciferous vegetables like broccoli. So **broccoli does double-duty: it helps balance estrogen and progesterone.**

Moreover, maintaining stable blood sugar levels through a balanced diet can indirectly support progesterone production. Consuming complex carbohydrates, such as whole grains, legumes, and nuts, rather than refined sugars, can help prevent insulin spikes. An animal study in 2021 highlighted the importance of **lowering refined carb intake for progesterone regulation**.[222] This suggests with falling progesterone levels after menopause you would not want to choose a diet rich in refined carbs.

A 2015 study showed omega-3 fatty acid supplementation increased progesterone levels in women with polycystic ovary syndrome (i.e. no cycle).[223] If you know any women

the *National Academy of Sciences of the United States of America.* 1997;94(25):14138-14143. doi:10.1073/pnas.94.25.14138

[222] Bishop CV, et al. Individual and combined effects of 5-year exposure to hyperandrogenemia and Western-style diet on metabolism and reproduction in female rhesus macaques. *Hum Reprod.* 2021;36(2):444–54.

[223] Rafraf M, et al. Omega-3 fatty acids improve glucose metabolism without effects on obesity values and serum visfatin levels in women with

with PCOS, they might eat more walnuts, chia seeds and flaxseed.

Additionally, Omega-3 fatty acids have been associated with enhanced insulin sensitivity and decreased available testosterone. In fact, you can **balance all three sex hormones with omega 3s.** Another study on 34 women showed available testosterone was significantly reduced after omega 3 supplementation with no change in SHBG. [224] Researchers observed no adverse effects on estrogen.

While these dietary changes may have a positive impact on progesterone levels, individual variations and underlying health conditions should be considered. Please note Vitamin B6 and magnesium are shown to help progesterone in cycling women. They are not reviewed here for postmenopausal women.

Research shows eating plant-based balances hormones. Women interested in details of a plant-based diet also shown to reduce the risk of lethal diseases like heart disease and cancer, are referred to *The Whole Foods Diet for Longevity*. Combining this dietary approach with intermittent fasting can further support weight management by balancing hormones.

Other nutrients for women's health over 50

According to Johns Hopkins medicine, you might also

---

polycystic ovary syndrome. J Am Coll Nutr. 2012 Oct;31(5):361-8. doi: 10.1080/07315724.2012.10720443.

[224] Phelan N, et al. Hormonal and metabolic effects of polyunsaturated fatty acids in young women with polycystic ovary syndrome: results from a cross-sectional analysis and a randomized, placebo-controlled, crossover trial. Am J Clin Nutr. 2011 Mar;93(3):652-62. doi: 10.3945/ajcn.110.005538.

ensure adequate vitamin D and calcium intake. You can optimize vitamin D via sunlight or supplements for improved hormonal balance.[225] Vitamin D deficiency in postmenopausal women is associated with increased risk of metabolic syndrome, joint pain, and possible bone fractures from osteoporosis.[226]

Johns Hopkins recommends 1.2g of calcium each day. The Osteoporosis Foundation states calcium rich foods include leafy green vegetables, broccoli, kale, beans, and almonds.[227]

Please note **for menopausal women, ensuring adequate vitamin D, calcium, and isoflavones is reported to improve body fat, hot flashes, anxiety, depressive symptoms, and sex life.**[228] So to combat symptoms after menopause you can also increase vitamin D and calcium, along with phytochemicals in plant foods.

Do you know an obese woman over 50 with cardiovascular disease? One 2018 study showed increasing iron reduced arterial stiffness by improving vascular endothelium

[225] Staying healthy after menopause. Johns Hopkins Medicine. Published August 8, 2021. https://www.hopkinsmedicine.org/health/conditions-and-diseases/staying-healthy-after-menopause#:~:text=Nutrition%20after%20menopause&text=After%20menopause%2C%20you%20should%20have,your%20risk%20of%20spinal%20fractures.

[226] Ko SH, Kim H. Menopause-Associated Lipid Metabolic Disorders and Foods Beneficial for postmenopausal women. *Nutrients*. 2020;12(1):202. doi:10.3390/nu12010202

[227] Bone Health and Osteoporosis Foundation. A Guide to Calcium-Rich Foods - Bone Health & Osteoporosis Foundation. Bone Health & Osteoporosis Foundation. Published May 20, 2020. https://www.bonehealthandosteoporosis.org/patients/treatment/calciumvitamin-d/a-guide-to-calcium-rich-foods/

[228] Ko SH, Kim H. Menopause-Associated Lipid Metabolic Disorders and Foods Beneficial for postmenopausal women. *Nutrients*. 2020;12(1):202. doi:10.3390/nu12010202

dysfunction.[229] Harvard will tell you foods rich in nonheme iron are plant foods like nuts, seeds, beans and lentils, and leafy green vegetables, e.g. spinach.[230] She could improve her cardiovascular disease by eating nonheme iron foods (i.e. plant foods).

Proper nutrition plays a significant role in hormone balancing. To optimize estrogen you want plant foods rich in fiber, omega 3s, and antioxidants like broccoli, nuts and seeds. Same goes for progesterone and insulin. For these you also want to replace refined carbs with whole food carbs high in fiber like berries, whole grains, beans, and seeds. Remember that you balance your hormones for optimal weight and performance when you eat plant-based.

In Chapter 5 you will discover real success stories with real women and working definitions for proven methods of weight loss. In Chapter 6 you will discover proven fasting plans for weight loss after menopause and more tips and insights for maximum weight loss in minimum time.

---

[229] Szulinska, M.; Loniewski, I.; Skrypnik, K. Multispecies Probiotic Supplementation Favorably Affects Vascular Function and Reduces Arterial Stiffness in Obese Postmenopausal Women-A 12-Week Placebo-Controlled and Randomized Clinical Study. *Nutrients* **2018**, *10*, 1672.
[230] Iron. The Nutrition Source. Published March 7, 2023. https://www.hsph.harvard.edu/nutritionsource/iron/ For more on iron see Chapter 2 in *The Whole Foods Diet for Longevity*

Chapter 5

Fasting Success Stories and Insights to Make Fasting Easier

Weight Loss Success with Real Women

We've seen amazing weight loss and health benefits from fasting research in Chapters 1-3. Before we review fasting protocols, how about a real, impressive, lasting result with a real woman? Here are three real results.

Marina was fighting breast cancer and fatty liver disease when she found Dr. Fung in 2018.[231] She was expecting a diabetes diagnosis. She failed multiple times to lose weight by following her doctor's advice to eat six small meals a day, join a gym, etc. She joined Dr. Fung's online community to stay on track with IF. **Marina lost 50 lbs while reversing much of her disease with one meal a day.**

Three strategies helped her lose 50 lbs. First, she was drinking water during fasting. She stayed hydrated. Second, she made herself busy to pay less attention to hunger which mitigated cravings for food. Lastly, she ignored social media, shopped less for groceries, cooked less, and avoided theaters and parties where people socialize with food. This helped not feed her hunger craving to not break her scheduled fasts. She may have cooked ahead of time and asked loved ones to go out or take food elsewhere to not be tempted to eat during

---

[231] Jason Fung. Intermittent Fasting Tips (My Top 3 Tips 2021) | Jason Fung. *YouTube*. Published online December 27, 2020. https://www.youtube.com/watch?v=W96LOxnlwTw

her fasts. Marina lost 50 lbs eating one meal a day.

Sarah lost over 80 lbs with intermittent fasting (IF).[232] She struggled with her weight for life by following advice like "everything in moderation." It failed. **Her secret to weight loss success was varying her eating windows via time-restricted feeding.** She started eating all food in eight hours a day (16:8) adding one day a week of fasts near 24 hours. Once a month she threw in a 36 hour fast, keeping her body guessing. **She lost over 80 lbs by varying her eating windows with time-restricted feeding.**

Debra lost almost 40 lbs with IF at 52 years of age.[233] Counting calories never worked. **With fasting she was sleeping better, her mood stabilized, and she reduced her blood pressure medication. She lost nearly 40 lbs** starting with skipping breakfast, building up to 16:8 and progressed towards one meal a day. She says fasting with her husband made it so much easier.

If these women can lose over 40 lbs with intermittent fasting, so can you! Here are some tips to help you get started.

Tips for beginners

A supportive environment can facilitate long term success with intermittent fasting. One 2009 study on 62 women

---

[232] Jason Fung. Intermittent fasting: fad or future? | Jason Fung. *YouTube*. Published online December 20, 2020. https://www.youtube.com/watch?v=CrsqleXWa6Y
[233] Jason Fung. Intermittent Fasting for Women | Jason Fung ft. Megan Ramos. *YouTube*. Published online March 28, 2021. https://www.youtube.com/watch?v=09YXEgMheE0 at 10:20

showed group support over six months yielded greater weight loss, more activity, and decreased binge eating.[234]

You could ask a friend or your spouse to keep you accountable and help identify your triggers and emotional eating habits (see below). As Debra said, fasting with her husband made it much easier to lose 40 lbs. Consider joining online communities or support groups where you can connect with like-minded individuals who are also practicing intermittent fasting.[235] Share your experiences, seek advice, and celebrate milestones together.

Remember what gets measured gets managed. In addition to stepping on your scale each week, you can use technology to tell you when you're burning fat. One affordable tool to measure whether you are in ketosis is the Keto-Mojo.[236] It measures ketones and blood glucose.

Many women who succeed with fasting keep a journal and use an app to track their fasting hours, food choices, and how they feel during different stages of fasting, e.g. Zero Longevity Science app. This data can help you identify patterns, understand your body's response, and make informed decisions to adjust your behavior for success. It is essential to listen to your body and adjust as needed.

---

[234] Tapper K, et al. Exploratory randomised controlled trial of a mindfulness-based weight loss intervention for women. Appetite. 2009 Apr;52(2):396-404. doi: 10.1016/j.appet.2008.11.012.
[235] For more info see TheFastingMethod.com
[236] Amazon.com: KETO-MOJO GK+ Bluetooth Glucose & Ketone Testing Kit + Free APP for ketosis & diabetes management. 20 blood test strips (10 each), meter, 20 lancets, lancing device, and control solutions : Health & Household. https://www.amazon.com/KETO-MOJO-%CE%B2-Ketone-Monitoring-Solutions-Ketogenic/dp/B08G5BZQVL

A study in 1990 found significant associations between levels of emotional eating and weight loss success. Research shows weight loss failure was associated with increases in emotional eating over one year and vice versa.[237] In other words, weight loss long term is associated with lower emotional eating. If you are eating when bored, stressed, or sad or overeating in response to the smell or flavor, you are eating for pleasure. That will not help with fasting goals.

By prioritizing a supportive environment, measuring progress, adjusting fasting as needed, and building healthy eating habits, you can enjoy long term success with intermittent fasting.

Mastering emotional eating

Now that you know science proves IF works for lasting weight loss, and countless other health benefits, does that mean you will do it? If we're being honest, maybe not. You can know something works and still not do it. If you master your emotions that cause you to eat, you will succeed faster and easier with fasting.

Research suggests weight regain within five years of weight loss is a result of the individual failing to maintain healthy eating and exercise habits.[238] Simply knowing *how* to lose weight is not sufficient. **For lasting success, we also**

----

[237] Blair AJ, Lewis VJ, Booth DA. Does emotional eating interfere with success in attempts at weight control? Appetite. 1990 Oct;15(2):151-7. doi: 10.1016/0195-6663(90)90047-c.
[238] Tapper K, et al. Exploratory randomised controlled trial of a mindfulness-based weight loss intervention for women. Appetite. 2009 Apr;52(2):396-404. doi: 10.1016/j.appet.2008.11.012.

need to change our psychology behind our weight gain habits.

Have you ever eaten when you're sad, hurt, or angry? Do you have a habit of snacking before and after dinner? Nowadays many women eat for pleasure or for flavor regardless of hunger. If you are eating when you're not hungry, outside your scheduled eating window, you are eating to change how you feel.

A lot of our decisions are based on emotions and we use logic and reason to justify them. If you are eating when you're not hungry or scheduled to eat, e.g. snacking, you are eating based on emotion. We even have a name for it: comfort foods. To not eat during your fasting periods, you MUST find an alternative behavior to replace the unhealthy snacking that makes you feel good.[239] For the alternative to be a permanent replacement, it will have to make you feel as good as the snacking. Maybe when you are feeling sad you replace eating ice cream or cheese(cake) by going for a walk by the water or going to the spa, as these also make you feel good by increasing dopamine levels in the brain. Maybe when you are fasting and you crave the flavor of ice cream or cookies you replace comfort foods with feeling love by talking to a close friend or family member, or feeling productive doing work. Whatever you do, you don't want to feed the craving.

Conquering food cravings

Good news! Science shows the more days you fast, the lower the food cravings. Food cravings occur in up to 97% of the

---

[239] Women interested in mastering emotions and changing behavior to feel great are referred to the most proven strategies in Robbins T. *Awaken the Giant Within: How to Take Immediate Control of Your Mental, Emotional, Physical & Financial Destiny!*; 1991.

population. A 2006 study in the journal *Obesity* showed that the cravings go down the longer you fast (the very low calorie diet in the study simulated fasting).[240] It gets better: it doesn't matter whether you crave carbs or high fat foods or sweet desserts. The cravings go down when you do not feed them. This result is similar to when your kids had chickenpox and you encouraged them not to scratch it. It is empowering to know the more you fast over time, the more it will lower food cravings. This will help you achieve your fasting goals even faster.

Avoiding environmental triggers

Do you know your triggers? Have you ever eaten in a meeting when you were not hungry because there was a plate of donuts on the table? If that plate of food was not there, you would not have eaten because there would have been no trigger for the eating.

Your environment can trigger you to eat when you're not hungry or scheduled to eat. Maybe you stop for a coffee every morning before work. Have you noticed the enticing pastries, muffins, cookies, etc. at the cash register? That may trigger you to eat a dessert when you otherwise would not. Also, desserts can make you feel pleasure even though you know they're bad for you. To avoid these triggers during your fasting periods you might decide to brew your own coffee in the morning instead of going to Starbucks. If there's no food for you to see and smell, there's no trigger to eat.

_____

[240] See figure 2 in Martin CK, O'Neil PM, Pawlow LA. Changes in Food Cravings during Low-Calorie and Very-Low-Calorie Diets*. *Obesity*. 2006;14(1):115-121. doi:10.1038/oby.2006.14

During your fasts you may want to avoid grocery stores, restaurants, or parties that will tempt you with food. You might also avoid social media during your fasting hours as there could be tantalizing pictures and descriptions of food. If you can think of any other food triggers during your day you would want to avoid them as well. If you can't think of any, maybe you could ask friends and family if they have observed any other triggers in your eating habits.

By now I hope you've decided to make intermittent fasting part of your lifestyle, using these hacks to make it easier for you. Below we'll define proven methods for weight loss.

Time-Restricted Feeding (TRF)

Time-restricted feeding involves restricting the daily eating window to a specific period while fasting for the remaining hours. This approach is flexible and can be adapted to your preferences and schedule. Popular options include 16:8, 14:10, or even shorter eating windows like 18:6. If you eat all food in six hours a day (18:6) you can repair and rejuvenate tissue with autophagy (see Chapter 2).

Fasting for 16 hours and limiting the eating window to eight hours each day is the most popular method (16:8). This approach is easily integrated into daily routines and you get to decide which eight hours to eat are most convenient for you. By skipping breakfast and having the first meal later in the morning or early afternoon, followed by another meal within the eating window, you can effectively practice 16:8. This way when you're eating nothing changes (i.e. one meal every 3-4 hours as usual).

To implement 16:8 fasting, choose a suitable eating window

that aligns with your lifestyle. For example, you may decide to have your first meal at noon and finish eating by 8pm, thereby fasting from 8pm to 12pm the next day.

Please note IF is not recommended for type 1 diabetics or a BMI under 18.5.

Alternate-Day Fasting (ADF)

Alternate-day fasting involves alternating between fasting days and non-fasting days. Fasting days could be water only while eating days are normal eating. On fasting days you may add herbal or green tea (zero calorie) beverages if you feel hungry.

This is key: during the eating window you are not trying to eat larger meals or whatever you want. You are just eating normal-sized meals as you always did about four hours apart. You are not going to feel successful and see weight loss if you try to eat six meals on your eating day to make up for eating zero meals on your fasting day.

According to Dr. Longo, ADF is more easily tolerated than calorie counting and provokes similar body composition and heart health benefits.[241] It's also proven safe for a period of over six months. **You heard that right! It's proven healthy to eat every other day for six months.** His extensive fasting research shows improved fat mass and cardiovascular disease risk factors after only four weeks of ADF. He wrote "ADF as a lifestyle intervention, could eventually accommodate modern healthcare practice."

---

[241] Longo VD, et al. Intermittent and periodic fasting, longevity and disease. *Nature Aging*. 2021;1(1):47-59. doi:10.1038/s43587-020-00013-3

Fasting-Mimicking Diet (FMD)

Dr. Longo is credited with creating this periodic fasting method. FMD is a plant-based periodic fasting method characterized by low protein and high unsaturated fats.[242] It was developed to mimic many of the benefits induced by water only fasting but with reduced side effects like hunger and hypoglycemia.[243] It is considered safe and easier for sick and bedridden people.

FMD would involve periods of two to seven days a month where you eat 300 - 1100 calories per day. The most common approach would be 500 calories for five days in a row each month. Dr. Longo does FMD twice a year for longevity benefits despite being in good health.[244]

Please note although FMDs appear to be safe, Dr. Longo says their use should be limited to three times per year in healthy people with normal levels of disease risk factors, until proven in longer term clinical studies.[245]

Here is a summary of the fasting methods from this chapter. Weekly variations and personalized approaches for weight loss are covered in Chapter 6.

---

[242] Ibid. See also Salvadori G, Mirisola MG, Longo VD. Intermittent and periodic fasting, hormones, and cancer prevention. *Cancers.* 2021;13(18):4587. doi:10.3390/cancers13184587

[243] Longo VD, et al. Intermittent and periodic fasting, longevity and disease. *Nature Aging.* 2021;1(1):47-59.

[244] Robbins T, Diamandis PH. *Life Force: How New Breakthroughs in Precision Medicine Can Transform the Quality of Your Life & Those You Love.* Simon and Schuster; 2022. pg 290

[245] Longo VD, et al. Intermittent and periodic fasting, longevity and disease. *Nature Aging.* 2021;1(1):47-59. doi:10.1038/s43587-020-00013-3

Method of IF	Description
Time-restricted feeding (TRF)	Eating all calories in less than 12 hours a day, e.g. 15:9 is eating all food in 9 hours a day
Alternate-day fasting (ADF)	Eating all calories normally for a day alternated with a day of 0-500 calories
Fasting-mimicking diet (FMD)*	Eating 300-1100 calories for a few days a month, e.g. eat normally 3 weeks a month plus 500 calorie days five days a month

* Not recommended on a chronic basis for healthy women, but proven effective for ill and overweight women

Part 3: Fasting Plans for Women after Menopause

Chapter 6

Weekly Fasting Plans for Maximizing Weight Loss after Menopause

Once you're on the other side of menopause fasting gets so much easier.[246]

- *Mindy Pelz, DC, chiropractor, bestselling author of The Menopause Reset*

Remember the fasting variation in Dr. Fung's patient that lost over 80 lbs? That's the plan you want to model for lasting weight loss. Here is a chart to keep handy for definitions of the types of IF so you can be in the driver's seat when scheduling the weekly plans below to suit your lifestyle. The weekly plans for postmenopausal women are essentially varied TRF plans and modified 5:2 plans.

Table 1: Fasting Methods to promote women's health[247]

Type of Fasting	Schedule	Description
TRF	12-18 h fast/ 6-12 h eating period	Eat in 6–12 h per day, e.g. 16:8 is eating in 8h per day

---

[246] Mindy Pelz. Fasting for Women without A Cycle | Fasting For Women. *YouTube*. Published online January 28, 2022. https://www.youtube.com/watch?v=zsJTmok9LgA at 7:30

[247] Adapted from Longo VD, et al. Intermittent and periodic fasting, longevity and disease. *Nature Aging*. 2021;1(1):47-59. doi:10.1038/s43587-020-00013-3

OMAD	24h fast	Eat only dinner or only lunch
ADF	24 h fast / 24 h normal eating	Water only fasting every other day
5:2 plan	2 days fast or 500 cal / 5 days eating period	Alternation of 2 days of 0-500 calories with 5 days normal eating (around 2000 calories)

The key to consistently lose weight and keep it off is to vary your fasting schedule. **For best results, vary the number of hours you fast each week or each day and spend some whole days not fasting**. You must go in and out of your fat burning and sugar burning systems; flip the metabolic switch on and off (see Chapter 3). The easiest way would be to vary TRF periods. How about some proven weekly weight loss plans for women over 50? Here are some clinically proven weekly variations for women after menopause. We will review top tips for beginners before covering extended fasting methods.

The 5-1-1 plan (modified 5:2)

The 5-1-1 plan is recommended by Mindy Pelz, DC, a chiropractor, bestselling author, and YouTuber on fasting for women. She committed herself to learning about fasting as she went through menopause. The following plans are arranged from relatively easy to more difficult.

In a 5-1-1 week you will eat all your food in nine hours a day for five days (15:9).[248] The next day you extend the fast from 15 hours to 17-24 hours. The last day can break the extended fast by eating over a 12 hour period as usual. So on one day of this week you would eat three meals every four hours to switch from fat burning back to sugar burning. Then repeat this the next week, slowly increasing the extended fast day up to 24 hours. This will extend your time spent in fat burning mode. The key with this plan is to vary the 1-1 sequence of the days in the plan and the time intervals spent practicing TRF. For example, one week you might do the five days of TRF at 16:8 instead of 15:9.

For beginners it will take time to build up to fasting 17-20h, eating all food in 4-7h per day. This would repair and rejuvenate your tissue (aka autophagy). Studies where people were eating in a 4- to 6-hour window each day showed 3% weight loss, reduced body fat, and waist size in just two months.[249] If you want significant weight loss in a couple months, you would want to build up to 20 hour fasts.

When you decide you're ready to extend the fast to 24 hours it's called OMAD (one meal a day). The easiest OMAD approach is to eat all your food at dinner then break your fast the next day at dinner. This 24 hour fast will extend the time for fat burning (ketosis) and cell repair and rejuvenation (autophagy). OMAD can optimize your thinking, learning,

[248] Mindy Pelz. Fasting for Women without A Cycle | Fasting For Women. *YouTube*. Published online January 28, 2022.
https://www.youtube.com/watch?v=zsJTmok9LgA at 7:30
[249] Cienfuegos S, et al. Effects of 4- and 6-h Time-Restricted Feeding on Weight and Cardiometabolic Health: A Randomized Controlled Trial in Adults with Obesity. *Cell Metabolism*. 2020;32(3):366-378.e3. doi:10.1016/j.cmet.2020.06.018

and memory (see Chapter 2). It may also benefit your skin and hair. In 5-1-1 you may do OMAD just once a week.

The 4-2-1 plan

This plan is modified 5-1-1 for weight loss and also improves menopausal symptoms like hot flashes. [250] You would eat for nine hours a day for four days (15:9). This can be done simply by skipping breakfast. Then you eat normally for two days to burn sugar (i.e. 12 hour eating window). Then you can switch back to fat burning the last day by fasting up to 24 hours. This may be more difficult since the extended fasting day follows two normal eating days.

Then you repeat this plan varying the extended fast day. Perhaps the first time you fast 17 hours on that day. Then the next week 20 hours, and maybe a full 24 hours on the extended fast day on the third week.

You might be progressively shortening the four day TRF eating window as the weeks go by. As your hunger and cravings bottom out, you may switch from four days of 15:9 to 16:8 to 18:6. In other words, you might eat in nine hour windows the first week, eight hour eating windows on week 2, then six hour eating windows week 3.

Eventually, you may feel energized with longer fasts. The shorter your eating windows get and the more you vary them, the quicker you should see and feel results. Once four days of eating in six hours feels easier, you might switch to four days OMAD or you could try ADF for four days.

---

[250] Mindy Pelz. Fasting for Women without A Cycle | Fasting For Women. *YouTube*. Published online January 28, 2022. https://www.youtube.com/watch?v=zsJTmok9LgA at 7:30

Top tips for fasting beginners: HBVR

Based on clinical results with thousands of women, Dr. Fung recommends these tips for women new to fasting.[251] You can remember the tips as HBVR: hydrate, be busy, vary the TRF, and be realistic.

Hydrate

When you're just starting out you can do water only fasts or 500 calories to simulate the effects of a water fast (FMD). Remember to add a pinch of sea salt if you have headaches or feel dizzy, though these should subside within a couple weeks of fasting.[252] At the outset you might drink some low calorie beverages during the fasting hours: green tea, herbal tea, black coffee, or bone broth. Try not to add sugar and cream to your coffee as you want zero calorie beverages.

Green tea has catechins that can suppress hunger and increase metabolic rate, facilitating weight loss. A 2009 review of six studies showed green tea users lost 3.3 lbs.[253] The catechins in hot tea facilitate weight loss via increased fat oxidation and decreased appetite.[254] Further, the caffeine

---

[251] Jason Fung. Intermittent Fasting Tips (My Top 3 Tips 2021) | Jason Fung. *YouTube*. Published online December 27, 2020. https://www.youtube.com/watch?v=W96LOxnlwTw

[252] Jason Fung. Beginning fasting (What to expect) | Jason Fung. *YouTube*. Published online March 7, 2021. https://www.youtube.com/watch?v=k8AkF9_hLow at 0:55

[253] Hursel R, et al. The effects of green tea on weight loss and weight maintenance: a meta-analysis. Int J Obes (Lond). 2009 Sep;33(9):956-61. doi: 10.1038/ijo.2009.135.

[254] Chen IJ, et al. Therapeutic effect of high-dose green tea extract on weight reduction: A randomized, double-blind, placebo-controlled

increases adrenaline leading to more activity (i.e. burning more calories). However, it would be better to drink herbal tea (decaf) during afternoon fasting so the caffeine does not impact your sleep and weight loss (see below).

Be busy to ride the hunger waves

You will be designing your fasting lifestyle for any of the compelling reasons in Chapters 1-3. Initially your body will be adjusting to the new schedule and you will feel hungry in the early stages unless you keep busy and focus on activities instead of eating. Good news: the more hours into your fast, the less hungry you feel. Research shows that if you work through lunch, hunger hormone levels fall to baseline by 4pm whether or not you ate lunch.[255] This means if you focus on working through lunch, the initial hunger wave will subside within a couple hours. I can personally verify this as I often worked through lunch in the months of research and writing for this book, where the hunger vanished by 3pm.

You could also schedule a meeting during a common eating window and by the time the meeting ends go right back to work. By staying busy it will be easier to let the hunger pass over you like a wave.

Think of all the free time you can use when you are not taking up time on meal prep! You can clean out your closet, walk outside, walk the dog, read a book, take a gym class, etc. This might be time you could keep busy playing sports you

---

clinical trial. *Clinical Nutrition*. 2016;35(3):592-599. doi:10.1016/j.clnu.2015.05.003
[255] See Figure 2 in Natalucci G, et al. Spontaneous 24-h ghrelin secretion pattern in fasting subjects: maintenance of a meal-related pattern. *European Journal of Endocrinology*. 2005;152(6):845-850. doi:10.1530/eje.1.01919

used to love. Maybe you schedule a tennis match or pickleball or go for a power walk during the time you decide not to prepare, eat, and clean up a meal.

Vary the time-restricted feeding windows

You must vary TRF to encourage your body to maximize time spent in fat burning mode (ketosis). Remember this is how Sarah lost over 80 lbs building up from 16 to 24 hours of daily fasting (see Chapter 5). IF is also shown to convert white fat stores to brown fat which is easier to burn.[256] The mechanism is similar to that of cold plunges for weight loss as explained by Dr. Rhonda Patrick.[257]

Realistic expectations

Remember fasting is a marathon, not a sprint. The scientific trials in previous chapters showed compelling results within months. So you do not want to set yourself up for failure by expecting results within days or weeks. Remember, the compelling results you will get from fasting are achieved like a marathon, not a sprint.

Accountability partner

The last tip to consider may be the most important. If you are committed to succeeding long term with a new behavior,

---

[256] Li G, et al. Intermittent Fasting Promotes White Adipose Browning and Decreases Obesity by Shaping the Gut Microbiota. Cell Metab. 2017 Oct 3;26(4):672-685.e4. doi: 10.1016/j.cmet.2017.08.019.
[257] For more on fat loss and cold plunges see FoundMyFitness Topic - Cold exposure. FoundMyFitness. https://www.foundmyfitness.com/topics/cold-exposure-therapy#brown-adipose-tissue-activation

get someone to do it with you.[258] This is the whole concept behind gym classes. It's easier to do something difficult when you have a group of people who share your goals. If you don't want to join a group of strangers, ask a friend or your spouse to fast with you. If you go it alone and let yourself down, you let yourself down. It happens. However, **if you are fasting with a loved one and you break your fast you are letting them down. That feels WAY worse than letting yourself down.** If you have someone to keep you accountable, you have the highest probability for long term success.

Another good tip from Dr. Fung is to eat as usual after fasting. For example, with OMAD, do not try to overeat at dinner on day 2 because you skipped breakfast and lunch. Clinically, you would never be told to overeat. "You have to eat normally when you resume eating and not overeat."[259]

Clinically proven OMAD plan for women

Eating one meal a day (OMAD) gives you more time in fat burning mode. Most will fast from dinner the day before to dinner the next day. For more weight loss you could try a clinically proven OMAD approach with hundreds of women from Dr. Fung's clinic. They found some women have trouble losing desired weight fasting dinner to dinner. These

---

[258] Jason Fung. Quick Intermittent Fasting Tips (Advanced) | Jason Fung. *YouTube*. Published online February 21, 2021. https://www.youtube.com/watch?v=XY7VRYfgMHk
[259] Jason Fung. The biggest fasting mistake | Jason Fung. *YouTube*. Published online October 17, 2021. https://www.youtube.com/watch?v=r6vkEIeBj_E

women succeeded by alternating days with lunch one day then dinner the next.[260]

If eating only dinner every day is not working, you could switch to fasting from lunch to dinner instead of dinner to dinner. For example, Monday, Wednesday, and Friday you could eat lunch, and Tuesday, Thursday, and Saturday you could eat dinner. This will be more difficult as it requires skipping dinner, the meal usually taken with family and friends, but it will achieve your desired result. It works because it alternates between 16 hours of fasting and 30 hours of fasting.

The 36 hour superfast for weight loss

This is not for beginners. Once you incorporate increasing fasting windows into your lifestyle up to 24 hours as above, you could add this superfast. Remember from Chapter 3 the power of adding 36 hour fasts and the more you fast, the more hunger dissipates. You could add a 36 hour fast once a month to spend more hours in a row in fat burning mode. For example, you could eat dinner Tuesday, fast Wednesday, then eat Thursday morning (fasting from dinner Tuesday to breakfast Thursday).

This is hard to incorporate into your lifestyle because you're skipping dinner, the most social meal of the day, typically eaten with family or friends. Maybe you could add this in initially if you or your spouse is traveling for work. It might be easier to do if your kids are out of town, e.g. Spring Break or away in college. Ideally, you could do it with your spouse.

---

[260] Jason Fung. Intermittent Fasting for Women | Jason Fung ft. Megan Ramos. *YouTube*. Published online March 28, 2021. https://www.youtube.com/watch?v=09YXEgMheEo at 6:00

Once one 36 hour fast a month feels comfortable, you could do it twice a month, working your way up to the study protocol. For maximum weight loss, you could mimic the study, cycling between a normal eating day and 36 hour fast.[261] To do this eat a 12 hour normal day, then fast 36 hours, then 12 hour eating day, 36 hour fast, etc. for 30 days. This will naturally signal your body to burn maximum belly fat in 30 days.

Remember with TRF that the length of fasting required for your body to be in fat burning mode (ketosis) will not be the same for every woman. One woman might be in ketosis at 12 hours, others at 20 hours, but anyone would be burning fat at 36 hours of fasting. This forces the body to burn fat as fuel as it drops insulin, signaling no food, so the body burns only fat for energy. To measure your ketones and time in fat burning mode you can use the Keto-Mojo (see Chapter 4).

For a personalized, proven weight loss approach, you could vary your time in TRF weekly using 5-1-1 or 4-2-1, changing the length of the extended fasting day. Using the top tips above will help you stay on course. Once you are used to these methods you can vary the time windows, e.g. building up from eating nine hours a day to six hours a day (15:9 to 18:6). You can also switch to more fat burning and autophagy by extending the extended fast day to one meal a day. If you want more weight loss, you could add in a 36 hour superfast once a month. This is how Sarah lost over 80 lbs (see Chapter 5). On top of scheduling when you eat, to lose more weight make sure you get enough sleep.

---

[261] Stekovic S, et al. Alternate day fasting improves physiological and molecular markers of aging in healthy, non-obese humans. *Cell Metabolism*. 2019;30(3):462-476.e6. doi:10.1016/j.cmet.2019.07.016

Optimizing your sleep to lose more weight faster

There does not seem to be one major organ within the body, or process within the brain, that isn't optimally enhanced by sleep (and impaired when we don't get enough).

- *Dr. Walker, bestselling author of Why We Sleep*

Did you know inadequate sleep can cause weight gain? Research shows sleep duration is trending down significantly. One 2015 study showed the number of adults sleeping less than six hours a night increased 31%.[262] Blame digital devices, streaming and social media?

Sleeping over seven hours a night is associated with weight loss. A 2022 study involved 80 overweight people sleeping less than 6.5 hours a night.[263] The group sleeping 6.5 hours ate almost 300 more calories per day. The other group was asked to sleep about one hour longer each night. The group sleeping over seven hours tended to eat less; 150 calories less. This means longer sleep helps you eat less and lose weight.

The study found the group sleeping around 6.5 hours gained weight (+1 lb) while the group sleeping around 7.5 hours lost 2 lbs. There was no difference in calorie burning. This is a prime study showing if you average 7-8 hours of sleep it can facilitate weight loss. **If you routinely sleep under**

---

[262] Ford ES, Cunningham TJ, Croft JB. Trends in Self-Reported Sleep Duration among US Adults from 1985 to 2012. *Sleep.* 2015;38(5):829-832. doi:10.5665/sleep.4684

[263] Tasali E, et al. Effect of sleep extension on objectively assessed energy intake among adults with overweight in real-life settings. *JAMA Internal Medicine.* 2022;182(4):365. doi:10.1001/jamainternmed.2021.8098

seven hours and want to lose more weight faster, you could simply sleep over seven hours a night. This is free and powerful for your health.

You also want routine sleep times. A 2009 study showed unusual sleep times lead to weight gain for two reasons: higher insulin and lower leptin. People were studied when they were sleeping in alignment with their circadian clock and when they were not (simulating night shift work). This study measured higher insulin (higher blood sugar) from eating the exact same meal during the night versus daytime.[264] It also measured lower leptin in the misaligned group. Insulin is the fat storing hormone and leptin is the satiety hormone to signal you you're full. **This means people sleeping unusual hours would store more fat and feel hungrier from the same meal,** e.g. working at night and sleeping in daylight. Working late into the night or going to work hours before dawn is a proven method to gain weight.

Dr. Walker is the foremost sleep expert, neuroscientist and bestselling author of *Why We Sleep*. He has researched sleep for over 20 years and authored over 100 scientific studies about sleep. He says routinely sleeping less than seven hours reduces cognitive performance and less than six hours increases risk for diabetes and high blood pressure.[265] This means sleeping over seven hours lowers risk factors for death by heart disease. He also says "routinely sleeping less than

---

[264] Scheer FA, et al. Adverse metabolic and cardiovascular consequences of circadian misalignment. *Proceedings of the National Academy of Sciences of the United States of America.* 2009;106(11):4453-4458. doi:10.1073/pnas.0808180106
[265] Robbins T, Diamandis PH. *Life Force: How New Breakthroughs in Precision Medicine Can Transform the Quality of Your Life & Those You Love.* Simon and Schuster; 2022. pg 308

seven hours a night demolishes your immune system."[266] These are all concerns after menopause.

A study on over 2100 student doctors found more feelings of depression with irregular sleep times.[267] Since depression symptoms are higher after menopause, and you want to maintain a stable circadian rhythm, this is one more reason to ensure adequate sleep duration and quality.

To add longer sleep to your fasting schedule for weight loss and other benefits you would want to measure your sleep. What gets measured gets managed. One simple test if you get enough sleep is to see if you wake up on time without an alarm. If not, you are sleep deprived. Here are tips from Dr. Walker to ensure optimal sleep duration and sleep quality.[268]

Go to bed and wake up at the same time every day

Your brain expects consistency. If you sleep in on weekends, it goes against your biological clock. When you go against your circadian rhythm it can manifest disease and dysfunction. Per Dr. Walker, "it's really getting in lockstep with our biology's expectation because when you fight biology, you typically lose - and the way that you *know* you've lost is usually through disease and sickness."[269] The best way to choose your sleep time may be the answer to this question: **if you were alone on a desert island with no power, when would you go to sleep and wake up?** To

[266] Ibid

[267] Fang Y, et al. Day-to-day variability in sleep parameters and depression risk: a prospective cohort study of training physicians. *Npj Digital Medicine.* 2021;4(1). doi:10.1038/s41746-021-00400-z

[268] See Robbins T, Diamandis PH. *Life Force: How New Breakthroughs in Precision Medicine Can Transform the Quality of Your Life & Those You Love.* Simon and Schuster; 2022. pg 309 - 313

[269] Ibid. pg 311

align with your circadian clock further, turn off all light sources before bed to signal your brain it's time for melatonin release for sleep.

Schedule your eight hour sleep opportunity window to ensure you get seven hours

If you go to bed and wake up at the same time every day you will train your body to rest and fast in a regular time window (you are fasting all hours of sleep). For example, you could schedule your sleep window every day from 11pm - 7am. This allows you an eight hour window to average over seven hours, accounting for the time it takes to fall asleep and wakefulness to use the restroom, nightmares, etc. We know sleeping over seven hours a night helps lose weight and reduces heart disease risk. Accordingly, Dr. Walker says "I don't want to invite disease into my life earlier than it has to be there. I don't want to live a shorter life."[270] Amen.

Measure your sleep

Dr. Walker recommends Oura Ring to measure sleep duration and sleep quality. It measures your sleep duration, deep sleep, REM sleep, restlessness, and readiness to start your day. You could also use a WHOOP strap. These devices will measure the effects your actions have on sleep and help you make better decisions for more valuable sleep duration and quality. WHOOP strap doubles as an outstanding fitness tracker with an accurate heart rate monitor that could also help you measure your fat burning aerobic exercise (see Chapter 3).

Act for sleep quality

---

[270] Ibid. pg 312

Optimal sleep temperature is 67°F. Dr. Walker suggests avoiding alcohol to avoid fragmented sleep, and avoiding caffeine (coffee and tea) after noon. Dr. Walker says

> Caffeine has a quarter life of twelve hours which means if you have a coffee at noon, 25% of that caffeine is still in your brain at midnight... even if you fall asleep it can decrease your deep sleep up to 20%. [This could] age you about 12-15 years.[271]

Remember you may feel vitally energized from fasting and have trouble falling asleep (aka onset insomnia). Fasting raises adrenaline. If this happens to you make sure you relax before bed. To do so, turn off your screens.

According to Harvard your devices emit a lot of blue light that amps up your sympathetic tone, slowing melatonin release.[272] This fight or flight response is the opposite of what you want to sleep. Instead of your phone or tablet, you might read a paperback book or magazine, or take a bath with Epsom salts and lavender. Any other relaxing activities you can think of could also help you fall asleep much easier than your phone or tablet.

Sleeping over seven hours a night facilitates weight loss and improves mental performance, common issues after menopause. It also boosts happiness and immunity, and lowers risk factors for heart disease, the top cause of death. If you want to lose more weight fasting, enjoy peak

---

[271] Ibid. pg 312
[272] Harvard Health. Blue light has a dark side. Harvard Health. Published July 7, 2020. https://www.health.harvard.edu/staying-healthy/blue-light-has-a-dark-side

performance, and live longer, make sure you track your sleep and get over seven hours a night.

Conclusion

Throughout this book, we have explored a multitude of benefits of intermittent fasting for women over 50. We have seen how intermittent fasting can lose weight long term, balance hormones, enhance mental performance, prevent cancer, promote cardiovascular health, promote anti-aging and longevity, and reduce pain (see Chapter 2). Leading scientific research shows intermittent fasting is a powerful tool that can positively impact various aspects of women's health after menopause.

Never forget that fasting is the most convenient, proven, safe dietary intervention used for thousands of years. It's free and saves you time. It's simple to follow. As Dr. Fung says "The simplest rule of weight loss is just don't eat all the time. This is a simple rule you can explain in 30 seconds that says don't eat between this hour and this hour." For these reasons intermittent fasting can be used by anyone, anywhere, and it can be done anytime you choose.

It may help to review the fasting myths covered in the Introduction when you are just starting out. Many people may respond to your change in lifestyle with myths like "fasting will make you feel starved and cause you to gain weight." Remember that what causes starvation mode is calorie counting from restrictive diets, not fasting. In truth, while fasting you will let the hunger pass over you like a wave. The best tip to do this is to stay busy with important tasks during a typical eating window (see tips in Chapter 6).

After reading the real results with real women using fasting in this book, know that you, too, can experience the transformative benefits of intermittent fasting after menopause (see Chapter 5). To do so you will be implementing the tips and strategies outlined in this book. Be sure to manage stress as it is shown to increase belly fat which could work against your fasting plan (see Chapter 3).

Incorporating intermittent fasting into your lifestyle requires a shift in mindset and a commitment to self-care. It is essential to approach fasting with a focus on balancing your hormones, optimizing nutrition, and following your fasting routine daily, weekly, and annually (see Chapter 4). Of course, these windows of time to eat and not to eat will be chosen by you. By choosing the right fasting method, setting realistic goals, and listening to your body, you can embark on a fasting journey that aligns with your unique goals and preferences.

Keep in mind it is always easier to do something new with someone you love. Make sure you have an accountability partner to start fasting with you, someone that you don't want to let down, e.g. your spouse or a close friend (see Chapter 6). Motivate each other and celebrate your progress together. You can also seek support from an online fasting community as you embark on this empowering journey towards improved health and wellbeing. Remember, intermittent fasting is not just about losing weight and keeping it off; it is about maximizing your energy levels, nourishing your body, living healthier and longer, and unlocking your full potential.

I am excited to welcome you to a growing share of the population practicing intermittent fasting for weight loss, health, and anti-aging benefits. Remember that intermittent fasting is a flexible approach personalized to suit your lifestyle. It may take time to find the fasting method and schedule that works best for you. You will feel empowered, determined and flexible as you design your fasting lifestyle. Embrace the power of intermittent fasting and discover the remarkable benefits it can bring to your life. Wishing you success and fulfillment on your intermittent fasting journey!

Thank You

Thank you to you, the reader, for reading this book. It was written to save you months or years doing research on your own to gather only the most credible information on intermittent fasting after menopause for weight loss and countless other health benefits.

Hopefully, you found this helpful to you or women you love. Please feel free to share this book with friends and family. Your feedback and support is most appreciated. Please go here to leave your valuable review online:

amazon.com/review/create-review/?asin=B0CSFVYHZB

Your valuable review could help women you know with weight management and living healthy, long, and strong. It will also help me with future editions and upcoming books in this series.

Thank you for reading!

Printed in Great Britain
by Amazon

38203062R00079